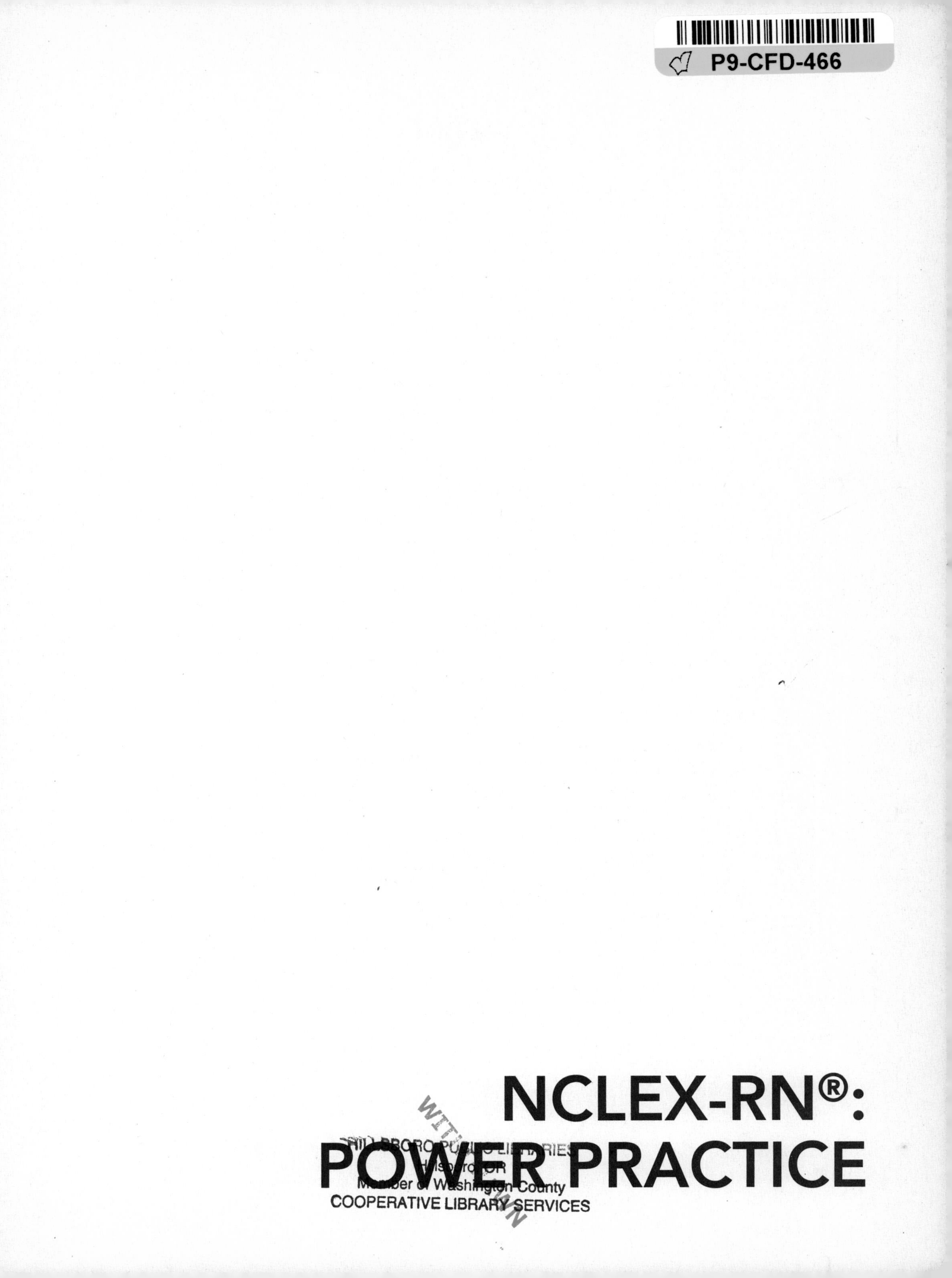

NCLEX-RN®: POWER PRACTICE

Related Title

NCLEX-RN Flash Review

NCLEX-RN®: POWER PRACTICE

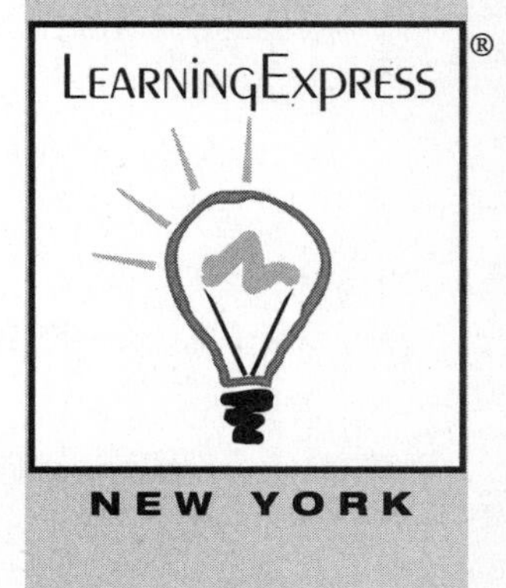

Published in the United States by LearningExpress, LLC, New York.

Library of Congress Cataloging-in-Publication Data:

NCLEX-RN : power practice.—1st ed.

p. ; cm.

ISBN 978-1-57685-908-7

I. LearningExpress (Organization)

[DNLM: 1. Nursing Care—Examination Questions. 2. Test-Taking Skills—Examination Questions. WY 18.2]

610.73076—dc23

2012032761

Printed in the United States of America

9 8 7 6 5 4 3 2 1

First Edition

ISBN-13: 978-1-57685-908-7

For more information or to place an order, contact LearningExpress at:

2 Rector Street
26th Floor
New York, NY 10006

Or visit us at:

www.learningexpressllc.com

CONTENTS

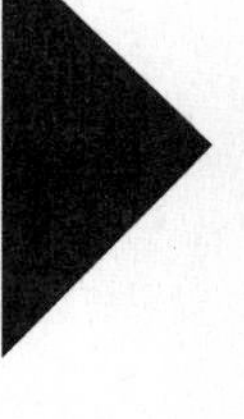

CONTRIBUTORS

Dr. Yvonne Weideman is an Assistant Professor of Nursing at Duquesne University School of Nursing. Her areas of interest are the preparation of students for the NCLEX exam and the use of innovative technology in the classroom to enhance learning. Dr. Weideman has recently developed a model for integrating theory and content through the use of virtual technology entitled "The Virtual Pregnancy Model."

Dr. Alicia Culleiton is an Assistant Clinical Professor at Duquesne University School of Nursing. She currently teaches doctoral-level nursing courses as well as undergraduate NCLEX-RN preparation courses. Dr. Culleiton earned her BSN from the Catholic University of America, her MSN in nursing administration and nursing education from Indiana University of Pennsylvania, and her doctorate from Chatham University. Her work has been published in nursing and educational journals. Her clinical expertise is in emergency/trauma and critical care nursing, with research interests that include student remediation and NCLEX-RN preparation.

Karen Paraska, PhD, CRNP, is assistant professor of nursing at Duquesne University. She has taught a range of graduate nursing courses that include offerings in advanced practice nursing and research methods, as well as undergraduate courses, including NCLEX-RN preparation courses. She is coauthor of several referred articles, including "Cognitive Impairment Associated with Adjuvant Therapy in Breast Cancer" for the journal *Psycho-Oncology*.

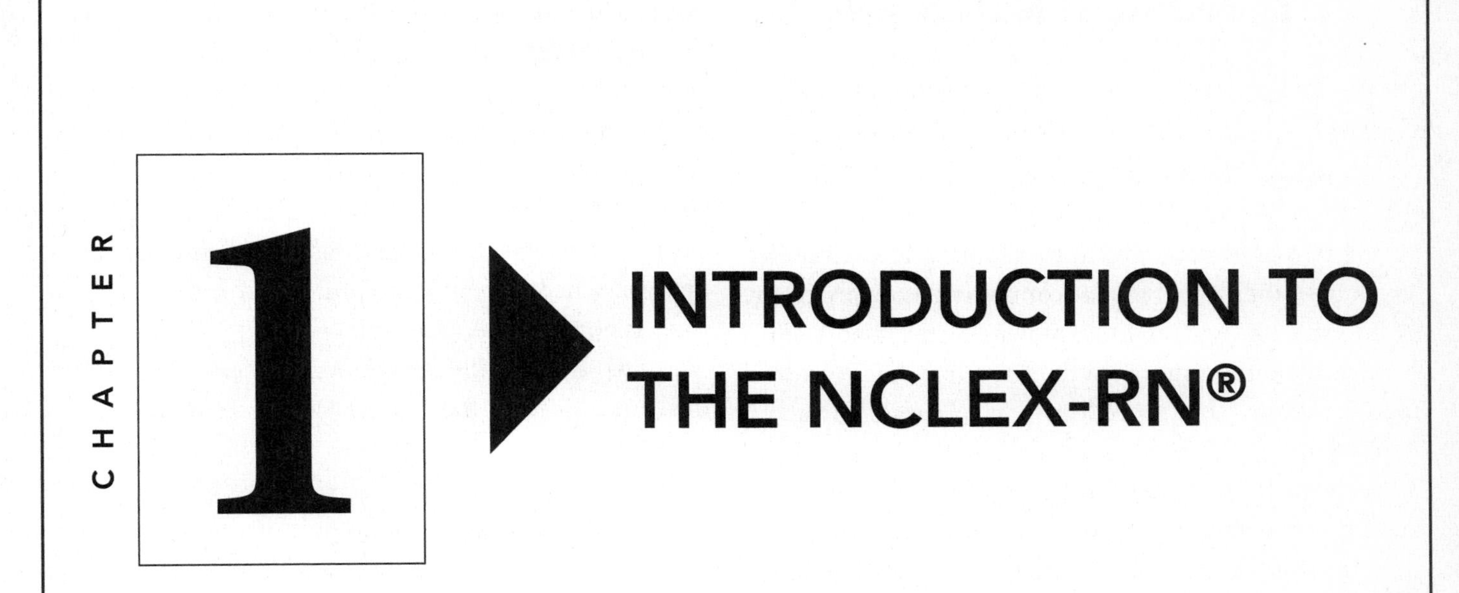

CHAPTER 1 INTRODUCTION TO THE NCLEX-RN®

Congratulations! If you are reading this book, it means that you have graduated or are about to graduate from an accredited registered nurse (RN) program and are interested in preparing for the National Council Licensure Examination for Registered Nurses (NCLEX-RN®) , which will enable you to gain a license as a registered professional nurse.

One of the most important ways to begin preparing for the NCLEX-RN is to become familiar with the format of the exam, the process of registering for the exam, what to expect on test day, the subjects the exam covers, and so on. This chapter will help you get started.

While the information in this chapter is current as of the date of publication, some details may change as time goes by. For the most recent information, refer to the official National Council of State Boards of Nursing (NCSBN) NCLEX website at https://www.ncsbn.org/nclex.htm.

Overview of NCLEX-RN

The NCLEX-RN is a computer-based exam that tests the knowledge, skills, and abilities you'll need to practice safely and effectively as an entry-level RN. The test is administered in a computerized adaptive testing (CAT) format, which, by adapting to each individual's abilities, allows the computer testing program to evaluate your abilities more effectively and efficiently than do more traditional approaches to testing. While the procedure the program uses is complex, the general principle is fairly simple. With each answer you record, the computer reassesses your competencies and continues to ask additional questions until it is virtually certain about whether your abilities are above or below the level required.

Given the test's adaptability, the number of questions it asks—anywhere from 75 to 265 items—is different for each individual. Of this number, 15 are pretest questions designed to help test producers develop new types of questions; these are not considered in your assessment. The exam is not divided into sections corresponding to content areas, though it is important that you understand what content areas are covered to help you prepare (see section "What Skills Are Tested?"). There is a time limit of six hours, no matter what number of questions you are given.

Registering for the Exam

Registration for the NCLEX-RN is a two-part process: applying for licensure with the board of nursing in the state or territory from which you are seeking your license, and registering for the exam with Pearson VUE, which administers the test. It is advisable to start both phases at once, so that both can proceed simultaneously.

You must meet all of your nursing board's requirements for taking the NCLEX-RN. (For a complete list of the boards of nursing and links to their websites, go to https://www.ncsbn.org/contactbon.htm.) The nursing board will certify to Pearson VUE that you are eligible to sit for the exam. This results in your Authorization to Test (ATT) letter, which must be shown the day of the exam. The ATT is valid for a time period—from 60 to 365 days—determined by your board of nursing, and the validity time frame cannot be extended. For this reason, it is important that you schedule your appointment for the exam as soon as possible after receiving your ATT.

Step-by-step, the registration process looks like this, as outlined in the "2012 NCLEX® Examination Bulletin":

1. Submit an application for licensure to the board of nursing where you wish to be licensed.
2. Meet all of the board of nursing's eligibility requirements to take the NCLEX.
3. Register for the NCLEX with Pearson VUE.
4. Receive Acknowledgement of Receipt of Registration from Pearson VUE.
5. The board of nursing makes you eligible to take the NCLEX.
6. Receive Authorization to Test (ATT) letter from Pearson VUE.
7. Schedule your exam with Pearson VUE.

Source: Taken from "2012 NCLEX® Examination Bulletin," page 2; available at https://www.ncsbn.org/2012_NCLEX_Candidate_Bulletin.pdf.

The fee to register for the exam is $200, which is nonrefundable. You must also pay a fee associated with the licensure application required by your nursing board. The registration is valid for a 365-day period, during which the nursing board will establish your eligibility. If a candidate doesn't meet the board's eligibility requirements within that time period, the registration fee is forfeited.

Failing to appear at the scheduled examination time will also result in both the forfeiture of your registration fee and the invalidation of your ATT, unless you reschedule one full business day before your scheduled time. If you don't pass the exam on your first try, you can retest based on a minimum waiting period—45 or 90 days—determined by your state nursing board.

More specific information about registration and scheduling can be found in the "2012 NCLEX® Examination Bulletin," available at https://www.ncsbn.org/2012_NCLEX_Candidate_Bulletin.pdf. This document and others found at the NCSBN's website should be checked to confirm details, which may change after publication of this book.

What to Expect at the Test Center

The NCLEX-RN is administered at one of the Pearson Professional Centers (PPCs); there are over 200 of them in the United States and 18 at locations outside the United States.

Plan to arrive at least 30 minutes before your test is scheduled to begin. Make sure to bring—in addition to your ATT letter—an acceptable personal form of identification (ID). The only IDs considered acceptable are a U.S. driver's license or U.S. state identification (both issued by your state's Department of Motor Vehicles), U.S. passport, and U.S. military identification. For test centers outside of the United States, only a U. S. passport is acceptable.

In addition to the ID you bring with you, other secure forms of identification will be taken during the check-in process, such as a digital signature and a palm vein scan. For further information on security procedures at the test site, refer to the "2012 NCLEX® Examination Bulletin," available at https://www.ncsbn.org/2012_NCLEX_Candidate_Bulletin.pdf.

During the Test

The test begins with a brief tutorial, during which you are instructed on how to use the computer you're working on. As you enter the testing room, the test administrator (TA) will give you an erasable note board with a marker, to be used for calculations and note taking. You cannot write on the note board until after the tutorial is finished; writing on it before is considered a serious violation and can result in an incident report and your results being placed on hold. If you need another note board during the test, you can raise your hand and ask the TA to provide you with one.

As mentioned, the time limit for the test is six hours. During that period there are two programmed optional breaks, one at two hours and another at three and one-half hours; the computer will inform you when these breaks start. You will also be allowed unscheduled breaks, such as those to use the restroom, but all breaks, including those that are scheduled, count against test time.

The testing environment is as standardized as possible to ensure that all candidates complete the exam under the same conditions. Strict controls, therefore, are in effect, such as the audio and video monitoring and recording and the restriction against cell phones, pagers, and other electronic devices in the testing room, as well as other personal items such as coats, hats, scarves, gloves, bags, purses, wallets, and watches. See page 8 in the "2012 NCLEX® Examination Bulletin," available at https://www.ncsbn.org/2012_NCLEX_Candidate_Bulletin.pdf, for more information.

What Skills Are Tested?

During the nursing program you have completed, much of your study was focused on specific areas of knowledge—such as anatomy and physiology, diseases and pathologies, and pharmaceuticals—needed to work as a registered nurse. The key to being an effective RN, however, is the application of that knowledge. Therefore, the questions—mostly multiple choice, though some in other formats—are designed to test whether you can apply that knowledge in the safe and effective care of clients as an entry-level RN. The exam, therefore, measures your understanding of the needs of clients you may encounter in practice, as well as your comprehension of the integrated processes critical in nursing to address these needs.

Client Needs

As mentioned, client needs compose the basic framework for the test plan. The client needs are broken down into four main categories, two of which have subcategories, as shown in the table.

Client Needs Categories	Percentage of Items in Each Category
Safe and Effective Care Environment	
Management of Care	16–22%
Safety and Infection Control	8–14%
Health Promotion and Maintenance	6–12%
Psychosocial Integrity	6–12%
Physiological Integrity	
Basic Care and Comfort	6–12%
Pharmacological and Parenteral Therapies	13–19%
Reduction of Risk Potential	10–16%
Physiological Adaptation	11–17%

Source: Taken from "2012 NCLEX® Examination Bulletin," page 13; available at https://www.ncsbn.org/2012_NCLEX_Candidate_Bulletin.pdf.

As explained next, these content areas cover the full range of ways that RNs are expected to attend to their clients' needs.

- *Safe and Effective Care Environment: Management of Care.* This content area addresses the ways in which nursing care should enhance the safety and effectiveness of the setting in which care is delivered and the ways that RNs must work to protect clients and healthcare personnel. The skills measured in this content area include, but are not limited to, advance directives, advocacy, case management, informed consent, and ethical practice.
- *Safe and Effective Care Environment: Safety and Infection Control.* This content area addresses the ways in which RNs should work to protect both clients and healthcare workers from health and environmental hazards. The skills measured in this content area relate to, but are not limited to, emergency response plans, handling hazardous and infectious materials, safe use of equipment, and use of restraints and safety devices.
- *Health Promotion and Maintenance.* This content area addresses the ways in which RNs should work to incorporate knowledge of growth and development principles, optimal health, and prevention and early detection strategies into the care of their clients. The skills measured in this content area relate to, but are not limited to, ante/intra/postpartum and newborn care, developmental stages and transitions, health promotion, disease prevention, lifestyle choices, and techniques of physical assessment.
- *Psychosocial Integrity.* This content area addresses the ways in which RNs should work to sustain and enhance the emotional, mental, and social well-being of clients as they undergo events causing stress as well as of clients dealing with acute or long-term mental illness. The skills measured in this content area relate to, but are not limited to, abuse and neglect, behavioral interventions, crisis intervention, end-of-life care, grief and loss, mental health concepts, and therapeutic communication and environment.
- *Physiological Integrity: Basic Care and Comfort.* This content area addresses the ways in which RNs should work to provide comfort to clients

and assist clients in performing activities and meeting expectations of daily living. The skills measured in this content area relate to, but are not limited to, assistive devices, elimination, mobility and immobility, nutrition and oral hydration, and rest and sleep.

- *Physiological Integrity: Pharmacological and Parenteral Therapies.* This content area addresses the ways in which RNs work to provide safe and effective care in the administration of medication and parenteral therapies. The skills measured in this content area relate to, but are not limited to, adverse effects, contraindications, side effects, interactions, blood and blood products, dosage calculation, expected actions or outcomes, medication administration, and parenteral/intravenous therapies.
- *Physiological Integrity: Reduction of Risk Potential.* This content area addresses the ways in which RNs work to reduce the likelihood of complications or problems that arise due to existing conditions, procedures, and treatments. The skills measured in this content area relate to, but are not limited to, vital signs, diagnostic tests, laboratory values, potential for complications of diagnostic procedures, and potential for complications from surgical procedures and health alterations, as well as system-specific (such as cardiovascular, endocrine, gastroenterological, integumentary, musculoskeletal, and neurological) assessments.
- *Physiological Integrity: Physiological Adaptation.* This content area addresses the ways in which RNs work to provide care, and to manage that care, for patients with acute, chronic, or life-threatening conditions. The skills measured in this content area relate to, but are not limited to, alterations in body systems, fluid and electrolyte imbalances, hemodynamics, medical emergencies, pathophysiology, and unexpected response to therapies.

For a more complete explanation and list of examples in each client need category, refer to the "2010 NCLEX-RN Detailed Test Plan, Candidate Version" (available at https://www.ncsbn.org/1287.htm).

Integrated Processes

Integrated processes critical to the practice of nursing are also addressed in the questions on the NCLEX-RN exam. These processes include all the methodologies employed by RNs in entry-level positions to address their clients' needs. As described in the "2010 NCLEX-RN Detailed Test Plan, Candidate Version" (available at https://www.ncsbn.org/1287.htm), they include:

- *Nursing process:* a scientific, clinical reasoning approach to client care that includes assessment, analysis, planning, implementation, and evaluation.
- *Caring:* interaction of the nurse and client in an atmosphere of mutual respect and trust. In this collaborative environment, the nurse provides encouragement, hope, support, and compassion to help achieve desired outcomes.
- *Communication and documentation:* verbal and nonverbal interactions between the nurse and the client, the client's significant others, and the other members of the healthcare team. Events and activities associated with client care are validated in written and/or electronic records that reflect standards of practice and accountability in the provision of care.
- *Teaching/learning:* facilitation of the acquisition of knowledge, skills, and attitudes promoting a change in behavior.

A Note on Guessing

Fast guessing may result in a drastically lowered score. In typical paper-and-pencil tests, and even some administered by a computer, unanswered items are marked wrong. But due to the nature of computerized adaptive testing, this strategy is ill-advised, since it will result in the computer program giving candidates easier items, which they may also get wrong if they are guessing and running short on time.

In short, rapid guessing should be avoided. You should simply maintain a steady pace, allotting approximately one to two minutes to each item; stay focused; and carefully read each item before answering.

Exam Results

Examination results are mailed—by the board of nursing—to the candidate approximately one month after the test. If you haven't heard after five weeks, you should contact your board of nursing, not Pearson VUE. Unofficial results are available within 48 hours through Quick Results Service for a small fee, if your board of nursing participates in the program.

To ensure quality and accuracy, the results are scored twice—once by the computer and a second time after the computer results are transmitted to Pearson VUE's central office. And even though the computer obtains the candidate's result, this information is not available to the test center's staff.

If you fail the exam, you will receive a Candidate Performance Report (CPR) from your nursing board. In addition to notifying the candidate of the unacceptable performance on the test, the CPR includes information about the number of items administered and the candidate's relative strengths and weaknesses vis-à-vis the test plan. With this information, the candidate will be guided in preparation for a re-examination. As mentioned, the retake waiting period depends on your board of nursing, and there will be a minimum of 45 or 90 days between exams.

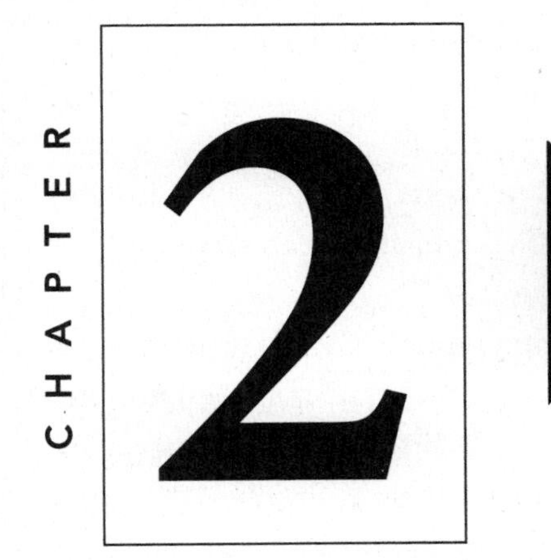

THE LEARNINGEXPRESS TEST PREPARATION SYSTEM

It takes significant preparation to score well on any exam, and the NCLEX-RN® is no exception. The LearningExpress Test Preparation System, developed by experts exclusively for LearningExpress, offers a number of strategies designed to facilitate the development of the skills, disciplines, and attitudes necessary for success.

Preparing for and attaining a passing score on the NCLEX-RN exam requires surmounting an assortment of obstacles. While some may prove more troublesome than others, all of them carry the potential to hinder your performance and negatively affect your scores. Here are some examples:

- lack of familiarity with the exam format
- paralyzing test anxiety
- leaving preparation to the last minute
- not preparing

- failure to develop vital test-taking skills like:
  - how to effectively pace through an exam
  - how to use the process of elimination to answer questions accurately
  - when and how to guess
- mental and/or physical fatigue
- test day blunders like:
  - arriving late at the testing facility
  - taking the exam on an empty stomach
  - not accounting for fluctuations in temperature at the testing facility

The common thread among these obstacles is control. Although a host of pressing, unanticipated, and sometimes unavoidable difficulties may frustrate your preparation, there remain some proven, effective strategies for placing yourself in the best possible position on exam day. These strategies can significantly improve your level of comfort with the exam, offering you not only the confidence you'll need, but also, and perhaps most importantly, a higher test score.

The LearningExpress Test Preparation System helps to put you in greater control. Here's how it works. Separated into eight steps, the system heightens your confidence level by helping you understand both the exam and your own particular set of test-taking strengths and weaknesses. It will help you structure a study plan, practice a number of effective test-taking skills, and avoid mental and physical fatigue on exam day. Each step is accompanied by an activity.

While the following list suggests an approximate time for the completion of each step, these are only guidelines for your initial introduction. The regular practice of a number of them may require a more substantial time commitment. It may also be necessary and helpful to return to one or more of them throughout the course of your preparation.

Step 1. Get information	1 hour
Step 2. Conquer test anxiety	20 minutes
Step 3. Make a plan	20 minutes
Step 4. Learn to manage your time	10 minutes
Step 5. Learn to use the process of elimination	20 minutes
Step 6. Reach your peak performance zone	10 minutes
Step 7. Make final preparations	10 minutes
Step 8. Make your preparations count	10 minutes
Total	2 hours, 40 minutes

We estimate that working through the entire system will take you approximately three hours. It's perfectly okay if you work at a faster or slower pace. It's up to you to decide whether you should set aside a whole afternoon or evening to work through the LearningExpress Test Preparation System in one sitting, or break it up and do just one or two steps a day for the next several days.

Step 1: Get Information

Time to complete: 1 hour
Activities: Read Chapter 1, "Introduction to the NCLEX-RN"

Knowing more about an exam can often make it appear less daunting. The first step in the LearningExpress Test Preparation System is to determine everything you can about the type of information you will be expected to know on the NCLEX-RN, as well as how your knowledge will be assessed.

What You Should Find Out

Knowing the details will help you study efficiently and help you feel a sense of control. Here's a list of things you might want to find out:

- What skills are tested?
- How many sections are on the exam?
- How many questions are in each section?
- How much time is allotted for each section?
- How is the exam scored, and is there a penalty for guessing and wrong answers?
- Is the test a computerized test or will you have an exam booklet?
- Will you be given scratch paper to write on?

Answers to these questions are in Chapter 1 of this book and on the NCSBN's NCLEX-RN website.

Step 2: Conquer Test Anxiety

Time to complete: 20 minutes
Activity: Take the "Test Stress Quiz"

Now that you know what's on the test, the next step is to address one of the biggest obstacles to success: *test anxiety*. Test anxiety may not only impair your performance on the exam itself, but also keep you from preparing properly. In Step 2, you will learn stress management techniques that will help you succeed on your exam. Practicing these techniques as you work through the activities in this book will help them become second nature to you by exam day.

Combating Test Anxiety

A little test anxiety is a good thing. Everyone gets nervous before a big exam—and if that nervousness motivates you to prepare thoroughly, so much the better. Many athletes report pregame jitters that they are able to harness to help them perform at their peak. Stop here and answer the questions on the "Test Stress Quiz" to determine your level of test anxiety.

Stress Management before the Exam

If you feel your level of anxiety is getting the best of you in the weeks before the exam, here are things you can do to bring the level down:

- **Prepare.** There's nothing like knowing what to expect to put you in control of test anxiety. That's why you're reading this book. Use it faithfully, and you will be ready on test day.
- **Practice self-confidence.** A positive attitude is a great way to combat test anxiety. Stand in front of the mirror and say to your reflection, "I'm prepared. I'm confident. I'm going to ace this exam. I know I can do it." Record these messages on a recorder as well. As soon as negative thoughts creep in, drown them out with these positive affirmations. If you hear them often enough and you use the LearningExpress method to study for the NCLEX-RN, they will be true.
- **Fight negative messages.** Every time someone talks to you about how hard the exam is or how it is difficult to pass, think about your self-confidence messages. If the someone with the negative messages is you—telling yourself you don't do well on exams, that you just can't do this—don't listen. Turn on your recorder and listen to your self-confidence messages.
- **Visualize.** Visualizing success can help make it happen—and it reminds you of why you're doing all this work in preparing for the exam. Imagine yourself beginning the first day of your dream job.
- **Exercise.** Physical activity helps calm your body and focus your mind. Besides, being in good physical shape can actually help you do well on the exam. Go for a run, lift weights, go swimming—and exercise regularly.

TEST STRESS QUIZ

You need to worry about test anxiety only if it is extreme enough to impair your performance. The following questionnaire will provide a diagnosis of your level of test anxiety. In the blank before each statement, write the number that most accurately describes your experience.

0 = Never
1 = Once or twice
2 = Sometimes
3 = Often

___I have gotten so nervous before an exam that I simply put down the books and didn't study for it.
___I have experienced disabling physical symptoms such as vomiting and severe headaches because I was nervous about an exam.
___I have simply not showed up for an exam because I was scared to take it.
___I have experienced dizziness and disorientation while taking an exam.
___I have had trouble filling in the little circles because my hands were shaking too hard.
___I have failed an exam because I was too nervous to complete it.
___**Total: Add up the numbers in the blanks.**

Your Test Stress Score

Here are the steps you should take, depending on your score. If you scored:

- **Below 3,** your level of test anxiety is nothing to worry about; it's probably just enough to give you that little extra edge.
- **Between 3 and 6,** your test anxiety may be enough to impair your performance, and you should practice the stress management techniques in this section to try to bring your test anxiety down to manageable levels.
- **Above 6,** your level of test anxiety is a serious concern. In addition to practicing the stress management techniques listed in this section, you may want to seek additional, personal help. Call your community college and ask for the academic counselor or ask the counselor at your nursing school. Tell the counselor that you have a level of test anxiety that sometimes keeps you from being able to take the exam. The counselor may be willing to help you or may suggest someone else you should talk to.

Stress Management on Test Day

There are several ways you can bring down your level of stress and anxiety on test day. They'll work best if you practice them in the weeks before the exam, so you know which ones work best for you.

- **Breathe deeply.** Take a deep breath while you count to five. Hold it in for a count of one, and then let it out on a count of five. Repeat several times.
- **Move your body.** Try rolling your head in a circle. Rotate your shoulders. Shake your hands from the wrist.
- **Visualize again.** Think of the place where you are most relaxed: lying on the beach in the sun, walking through the park, or wherever relaxes you. Now, close your eyes and imagine you're actually there. If you practice in advance, you will find that you need only a few seconds of this exercise to experience a significant increase in your sense of relaxation and well-being.

When anxiety threatens to overwhelm you *during* the test, there are still things you can do to manage your stress level:

- **Repeat your self-confidence messages.** You should have them memorized by now. Say them quietly to yourself, and believe them!
- **Visualize one more time.** This time, visualize yourself moving smoothly and quickly through the exam, answering every question correctly, and finishing just before time is up. Like most visualization techniques, this one works best if you've practiced it ahead of time.
- **Find an easy question.** Skim over the questions until you find an easy one, and then answer it. Getting even one question answered correctly gets you into the test-taking groove.
- **Take a mental break.** Everyone loses concentration once in a while during a long exam. It's normal, so you shouldn't worry about it. Instead, accept what has happened. Say to yourself, "Hey, I lost it there for a minute. My brain is taking a break." Close your eyes, and do some deep breathing for a few seconds. Then go back to work.

Try these techniques ahead of time and see if they work for you!

Step 3: Make a Plan

Time to complete: 20 minutes
Activity: Construct a study plan

There is no substitute for careful preparation and practice over time. So the most important thing you can do to better prepare yourself for your exam is to create a study plan or schedule and then follow it. This will help you avoid cramming at the last minute, which is an ineffective study technique that will only add to your anxiety.

Once you have your plan, make a commitment to follow it. Set aside at least 30 minutes every day for studying and practice. This will do more good than two hours crammed into a Saturday. If you have months before the test, you're lucky. Don't put off your studying until the week before. Start now. Even 10 minutes a weekday, with half an hour or more on weekends, can make a big difference in your score.

Step 4: Learn to Manage Your Time

Time to complete: 10 minutes to read; many hours of practice
Activities: Practice these strategies as you take the sample exams

Steps 4, 5, and 6 of the LearningExpress Test Preparation System put you in charge of your NCLEX-RN experience by showing you test-taking strategies that work. Practice these strategies as you take the practice exams in this book and online. Then, you will be ready to use them on test day.

First, you will take control of your time on the NCLEX-RN. Start by understanding the format of the test. Refer to Chapter 1 to review this information; in particular, make sure you understand the way the computerized adaptive testing (CAT) works.

You will want to practice using your time wisely on the practice tests, while trying to avoid making mistakes at the same time as working quickly.

- **Listen carefully to directions.** By the time you get to the test, you should know how it works. But listen carefully in case something has changed.
- **Pace yourself.** Glance at your watch every few minutes to ensure that you are not taking much more than one to two minutes on each item.
- **Keep moving.** Don't spend too much time on one question. If you don't know the answer, skip the question and move on. Mark the question for review, and come back to it later.
- **Don't rush.** You should keep moving; but rushing won't help. Try to keep calm and work methodically and quickly.

Step 5: Learn to Use the Process of Elimination

Time to complete: 20 minutes
Activity: Complete worksheet on "Using the Process of Elimination"

After time management, the next most important tool for taking control of your test is using the process of elimination wisely. It's standard test-taking wisdom that you should always read all the answer choices before choosing your answer. This helps you find the right answer by eliminating wrong answer choices. Consider the following question. Although it is not the type of question you will see on NCLEX-RN, the mental process that you use will be the same.

9. **Sentence 6:** I would like to be considered for the assistant manager position in your company my previous work experience is a good match for the job requirements posted.
Which correction should be made to sentence 6?
a. Insert *Although* before *I*.
b. Insert a question mark after *company*.
c. Insert a semicolon and *However* before *my*.
d. Insert a period after *company* and capitalize *my*.
e. No corrections are necessary.

If you happen to know that sentence 6 is a run-on sentence and you know how to correct it, you don't need to use the process of elimination. But let's assume that, like some people, you don't. So, you look at the answer choices. *Although* surely doesn't sound like a good choice, because it would change the meaning of the sentence. So, you eliminate choice **a**—and now you have only four answer choices to deal with. Write **a** on your note board with an X through or beside it. Move on to the other answer choices.

If you know that the first part of the sentence does not ask a question, you can eliminate choice **b** as a possible answer. Write **b** on your note board with an X through or beside it. Choice **c**, inserting a semicolon, could create a pause in an otherwise long sentence, but inserting the capitalized word *However* might not be correct. If you're not sure whether this answer is correct, write **c** on your note board with a question mark beside it, meaning "well, maybe."

Answer choice **d** would separate a very long sentence into two shorter sentences, and it would not change the meaning. It could work, so write **d** on your note board with a check mark beside it, meaning "good answer." Answer choice **e** means that the sentence is fine like it is and doesn't need any changes. The sentence could make sense as it is, but it is definitely long. Is this the best way to write the sentence? If you're not sure, write **e** on your note board with a question mark beside it.

Now, your note board looks like this:

X a.
X b.
? c.
✓ d.
? e.

You've got just one check mark, for a good answer, **d.** If you're pressed for time, you should simply select choice **d.** If you've got the time to be extra careful, you could compare your check mark answer to your question mark answers to make sure that it's better. (It is: Sentence 6 is a run-on, and should be separated into two shorter, complete sentences.)

It's good to have a system for marking good, bad, and maybe answers. We recommend using this one:

X = bad
✓ = good
? = maybe

If you don't like these marks, devise your own system. Just make sure you do it long before exam day—while you're working through the practice tests in this book and online—so you won't have to worry about it during the exam.

Even when you think you're absolutely clueless about a question, you can use the process of elimination to get rid of one answer choice. By doing so, you're better prepared to make an educated guess, as you will see next. More often, the process of elimination allows you to get down to only two possible right answers. Nevertheless, as explained in Chapter 1, rapid guessing is a strategy that should be avoided in the NCLEX-RN. It will result in the computer program giving candidates easier items, which you may also get wrong if you are guessing and running short on time.

Try using your powers of elimination on the questions starting on page 14. The answer explanations show one possible way you might use the process to arrive at the right answer.

Step 6: Reach Your Peak Performance Zone

Time to complete: 10 minutes to read; weeks to complete!
Activity: Complete the "Physical Preparation Record"

Physical and mental fatigue can significantly hinder your ability to perform as you prepare and also on the day of the exam. Poor diet choices can, as well. Drastic changes to your existing daily routine may cause a disruption too great to be helpful, but modest, calculated alterations in your level of physical activity, the quality of your diet, and the amount and regularity of your rest can enhance your studies and your performance on the exam.

USING THE PROCESS OF ELIMINATION

Use the process of elimination to answer the following questions.

1. Ilsa is as old as Meghan will be in five years. The difference between Ed's age and Meghan's age is twice the difference between Ilsa's age and Meghan's age. Ed is 29. How old is Ilsa?
   a. 4
   b. 10
   c. 19
   d. 24

2. "All drivers of commercial vehicles must carry a valid commercial driver's license whenever operating a commercial vehicle."
   According to this sentence, which of the following people need NOT carry a commercial driver's license?
   a. a truck driver idling his engine while waiting to be directed to a loading dock
   b. a bus operator backing her bus out of the way of another bus in the bus lot
   c. a taxi driver driving his personal car to the grocery store
   d. a limousine driver taking the limousine to her home after dropping off her last passenger of the evening

3. Smoking tobacco has been linked to
   a. increased risk of stroke and heart attack.
   b. all forms of respiratory disease.
   c. increasing mortality rates over the past 10 years.
   d. juvenile delinquency.

4. Which of the following words is spelled correctly?
   a. incorrigible
   b. outragous
   c. domestickated
   d. understandible

Answers

Here are the answers, as well as some suggestions as to how you might have used the process of elimination to find them.

1. d. You should have eliminated choice **a** right off the bat. Ilsa can't be four years old if Meghan is going to be Ilsa's age in five years. The best way to eliminate other answer choices is to try plugging them into the information given in the problem. For instance, for choice **b**, if Ilsa is 10, then Meghan must be 5. The difference between their ages is 5. The difference between Ed's age, 29, and Meghan's age, 5, is 24. Is 24 two times 5? No. Then choice **b** is wrong. You could eliminate choice **c** in the same way and be left with choice **d**.

2. c. Note the word *not* in the question, and go through the answers one by one. Is the truck driver in choice **a** "operating a commercial vehicle"? Yes, idling counts as "operating," so he needs to have a commercial driver's license. Likewise, the bus operator in choice **b** is operating a commercial vehicle; the question doesn't say the operator has to be on the street. The limo driver in choice **d** is operating a commercial vehicle, even if it doesn't have a passenger in it. However, the driver in choice **c** is not operating a commercial vehicle, but his own private car.

USING THE PROCESS OF ELIMINATION (*CONTINUED*)

3. a. You could eliminate choice **b** simply because of the presence of the word *all.* Such absolutes hardly ever appear in correct answer choices. Choice **c** looks attractive until you think a little about what you know—aren't fewer people smoking these days, rather than more? So how could smoking be responsible for a higher mortality rate? (If you didn't know that mortality rate means the rate at which people die, you might keep this choice as a possibility, but you would still be able to eliminate two answers and have only two to choose from.) And choice **d** is plain silly, so you could eliminate that one, too. You are left with the correct choice, **a**.

4. a. How you used the process of elimination here depends on which words you recognized as being spelled incorrectly. If you knew that the correct spellings were *outrageous, domesticated*, and *understandable*, then you would be home free. Surely you knew that at least one of those words was wrong in the question!

YOUR GUESSING ABILITY

The following are ten really hard questions. You are not supposed to know the answers. Rather, this is an assessment of your ability to guess when you don't have a clue. Read each question carefully, as if you were expected to answer it. If you have any knowledge of the subject, use that knowledge to help you eliminate wrong answer choices.

1. September 7 is Independence Day in
a. India.
b. Costa Rica.
c. Brazil.
d. Australia.

2. Which of the following is the formula for determining the momentum of an object?
a. $p = MV$
b. $F = ma$
c. $P = IV$
d. $E = mc^2$

3. Because of the expansion of the universe, the stars and other celestial bodies are all moving away from each other. This phenomenon is known as
a. Newton's first law.
b. the big bang.
c. gravitational collapse.
d. Hubble flow.

4. American author Gertrude Stein was born in
a. 1713.
b. 1830.
c. 1874.
d. 1901.

5. Which of the following is NOT one of the Five Classics attributed to Confucius?
a. *I Ching*
b. *Book of Holiness*
c. *Spring and Autumn Annals*
d. *Book of History*

6. The religious and philosophical doctrine that holds that the universe is constantly in a struggle between good and evil is known as
a. Pelagianism.
b. Manichaeanism.
c. neo-Hegelianism.
d. Epicureanism.

7. The third Chief Justice of the U.S. Supreme Court was
- **a.** John Blair.
- **b.** William Cushing.
- **c.** James Wilson.
- **d.** John Jay.

8. Which of the following is the poisonous portion of a daffodil?
- **a.** the bulb
- **b.** the leaves
- **c.** the stem
- **d.** the flowers

9. The winner of the Masters golf tournament in 1953 was
- **a.** Sam Snead.
- **b.** Cary Middlecoff.
- **c.** Arnold Palmer.
- **d.** Ben Hogan.

10. The state with the highest per capita personal income in 1980 was
- **a.** Alaska.
- **b.** Connecticut.
- **c.** New York.
- **d.** Texas.

Answers

Check your answers against the following correct answers.

1. c.
2. a.
3. d.
4. c.
5. b.
6. b.
7. b.
8. a.
9. d.
10. a.

How Did You Do?

You may have simply gotten lucky and actually known the answer to one or two questions. In addition, your guessing was probably more successful if you were able to use the process of elimination on any of the questions. Maybe you didn't know who the third Chief Justice was (question 7), but you knew that John Jay was the first. In that case, you would have eliminated choice **d** and, therefore, improved your odds of guessing right from one in four to one in three.

According to probability, you should get two-and-a-half answers correct, so getting either two or three right would be average. If you got four or more right, you may be a really terrific guesser. If you got one or none right, you may be a really bad guesser.

Keep in mind, though, that this is only a small sample. You should continue to keep track of your guessing ability as you work through the sample questions in this book. Circle the numbers of questions you guess on as you make your guess; or, if you don't have time while you take the practice tests, go back afterward and try to remember which questions you guessed at. Remember, on a test with four answer choices, your chance of guessing correctly is one in four. So keep a separate "guessing" score for each exam. How many questions did you guess on? How many did you get right? If the number you got right is at least one-fourth of the number of questions you guessed on, you are at least an average guesser—maybe better—and you should always go ahead and guess on the real exam. If the number you got right is significantly lower than one-fourth of the number you guessed on, you would be safe in guessing anyway, but maybe you would feel more comfortable if you guessed only selectively, when you can eliminate a wrong answer or at least have a good feeling about one of the answer choices.

Remember, even if you are a play-it-safe person with lousy intuition, you are still safe guessing every time.

Exercise

If you are already engaged in a regular program of physical activity, resist allowing the pressure of the approaching exam to alter this routine. If you have not been engaged in regular physical activity, it may be helpful to begin during your test preparations. Speak with someone knowledgeable about such matters to design a regimen suited to your particular circumstances and needs. Whatever its form, try to keep it a regular part of your preparation as the exam approaches.

Diet

A balanced diet will help you achieve peak performance. Limit your caffeine and junk food intake as you continue on your preparation journey. Eat plenty of fruits and vegetables, along with lean proteins and complex carbohydrates. Foods that are high in lecithin (an amino acid), such as fish and beans, are especially good brain foods.

Your diet is also a matter that is particular to you, so any major alterations to it should be discussed with a person with expert knowledge of nutrition.

Rest

For your brain and body to function at optimal levels, they must have an adequate amount of rest. It will be important to determine what an adequate amount of rest is for you. Determine how much rest you must have to feel at your sharpest and most alert, and make an effort to get that amount regularly as the exam approaches and particularly on the night before the exam.

It may help to record your efforts. On page 18 is a "Physical Preparation Record" for the week prior to the exam; you may find its use helpful for staying on track.

Physical Preparation Record

In the week leading up to the test, you may be so involved with studying (and, unfortunately, stress) that you neglect to treat your body kindly. This worksheet will help you stay on track.

For each day of the week before the test, write down what physical exercise you engaged in and for how long and what you ate for each meal. Remember, you're trying for at least half an hour of exercise every other day (preferably every day) and a balanced diet that is light on junk food. These practices are key to your body and brain working at their peaks.

Step 7: Make Final Preparations

Time to complete: 10 minutes to read; time to complete will vary
Activity: Complete the "Final Preparations" worksheet

You're in control of your mind and body; you're in charge of test anxiety, your preparation, and your test-taking strategies. Now, it's time to take charge of external factors, like the testing site and the materials you need for taking the test.

Find Out Where the Exam Is and Make a Trial Run

Make sure you know exactly when and where your test is being held. Do you know how to get to the exam site? Do you know how long it will take to get there? If not, make a trial run if possible, preferably on the same day of the week at the same time of day. On the "Final Preparations" worksheet, make note of the amount of time it will take you to get to the test site. Plan on arriving at least 30 to 45 minutes early so

PHYSICAL PREPARATION RECORD

For the week before the test, record (1) the type and duration of your physical exercise, (2) your food consumption for each day, and (3) the number of hours you slept.

Exam minus 7 days

Exercise: ______ for ______ minutes

Breakfast: ____________________________________

Lunch: ____________________________________

Dinner: ____________________________________

Snacks: ____________________________________

Exam minus 6 days

Exercise: ______ for ______ minutes

Breakfast: ____________________________________

Lunch: ____________________________________

Dinner: ____________________________________

Snacks: ____________________________________

Exam minus 5 days

Exercise: ______ for ______ minutes

Breakfast: ____________________________________

Lunch: ____________________________________

Dinner: ____________________________________

Snacks: ____________________________________

Exam minus 4 days

Exercise: ______ for ______ minutes

Breakfast: ____________________________________

Lunch: ____________________________________

Dinner: ____________________________________

Snacks: ____________________________________

Exam minus 3 days

Exercise: ______ for ______ minutes

Breakfast: ____________________________________

Lunch: ____________________________________

Dinner: ____________________________________

Snacks: ____________________________________

Exam minus 2 days

Exercise: ______ for ______ minutes

Breakfast: ____________________________________

Lunch: ____________________________________

Dinner: ____________________________________

Snacks: ____________________________________

Exam minus 1 day

Exercise: ______ for ______ minutes

Breakfast: ____________________________________

Lunch: ____________________________________

Dinner: ____________________________________

Snacks: ____________________________________

you can get the lay of the land, use the bathroom, and calm down. Then figure out how early you will have to get up that morning, and make sure you get up that early every day for a week before the test.

Gather Your Materials

Make sure you have all the materials that will be required at the testing facility. Whether it's an admission ticket, an ID, a second form of ID, pencils, pens, or any other item that may be necessary, make sure you have put it aside. It's preferable to put them all aside together.

Arrange your clothes the evening before the exam. Dress in layers so that you can adjust readily to the temperature of the exam room.

Fuel Appropriately

Decide on a meal to eat in the time before your exam. Taking the exam on an empty stomach is something to avoid, particularly if it is an exam that spans several hours. Eating poorly and feeling lethargic are also to be avoided. Decide on a meal that will sate your hunger without adverse effect.

Final Preparations

To help organize your final preparations, a "Final Preparations" worksheet is provided on page 20.

Step 8: Make Your Preparations Count

Time to complete: 10 minutes, plus test-taking time
Activity: Ace the NCLEX-RN!

Fast-forward to test day. You're ready. You made a study plan and followed through. You practiced your test-taking strategies while working through this book. You're in control of your physical, mental, and emotional state. You know when and where to show up and what to bring with you. In other words, you're well prepared!

When you're done with the test you will have earned a reward. Plan a celebration. Call up your friends and plan a party, have a nice dinner with your family, or pick out a movie to see—whatever your heart desires.

And then do it. Go into the test, full of confidence, armed with test-taking strategies you've practiced until they're second nature. You're in control of yourself, your environment, and your performance on the exam. You're ready to succeed. So do it, and look forward to your future as someone who has passed the NCLEX-RN!

FINAL PREPARATIONS

Getting to the exam site:

Exam date: ______________________________

Location of exam site: ______________________________

Do I know how to get to the exam site? Yes ___ No ___ (If no, make a trial run.)

Time it will take to get to the exam site: ______________________________

Departure time: ______________________________

Things to Lay Out the Night Before

Clothes I will wear ___

Sweater/jacket ___

Watch ___

Photo ID ___

Four #2 pencils ___

Other Things to Bring/Remember

______________________ ______________________

______________________ ______________________

______________________ ______________________

______________________ ______________________

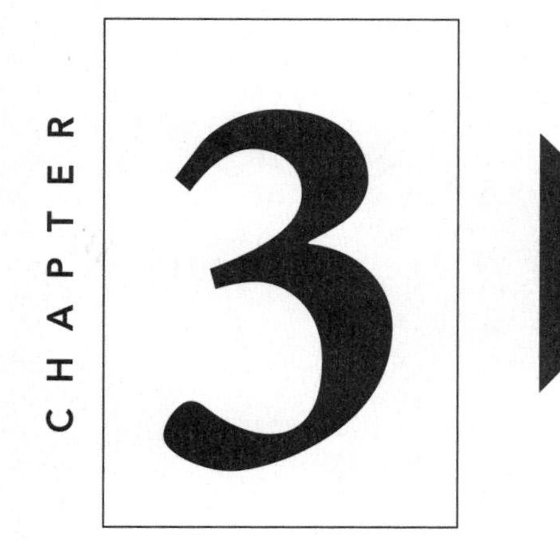

NCLEX-RN PRACTICE TEST 1

This examination has been designed to test your understanding of the content included on the National Council Licensure Examination for Registered Nurses (NCLEX-RN), which you must pass to become a registered nurse, and also to allow you to experience the format in which the exam is administered. Becoming comfortable with the examination format and logistics will help you be more relaxed when it comes to actually sitting for the test, enabling you to perform at your best.

The actual NCLEX-RN examination is computer adaptive, which means all examinees will have a different number of test questions depending on how many and what types of questions they answer correctly and how many they answer incorrectly. All test takers must answer a minimum of 75 items, and the maximum number of items that the candidate may answer is 265 during the allotted six-hour time period. This LearningExpress practice exam has 165 questions, and you should allow yourself four hours to complete it.

Then, after you have completed the exam, look at the answer key to read the rationales for both the correct and the incorrect choices, as well as the sources of the information. It is recommended that you utilize the sources to thoroughly review information that was problematic for you. Because the NCLEX-RN examination is graded on a sliding scale that is based on the difficulty of each particular exam, we are unable to predict how many correct answers would equate to an actual passing grade on this practice exam.

Completion of this examination represents the culmination of extensive test preparation. You have worked very hard to review the information from your NCLEX-RN curriculum, and now it is your time to shine. Good luck!

Practice Test 1 Answer Sheet

1. ⓐ ⓑ ⓒ ⓓ
2. ⓐ ⓑ ⓒ ⓓ
3. ⓐ ⓑ ⓒ ⓓ
4. ⓐ ⓑ ⓒ ⓓ
5. ⓐ ⓑ ⓒ ⓓ
6. ⓐ ⓑ ⓒ ⓓ
7. ⓐ ⓑ ⓒ ⓓ
8. ⓐ ⓑ ⓒ ⓓ
9. ⓐ ⓑ ⓒ ⓓ
10. ⓐ ⓑ ⓒ ⓓ
11. ⓐ ⓑ ⓒ ⓓ
12. ⓐ ⓑ ⓒ ⓓ
13. ⓐ ⓑ ⓒ ⓓ
14. ⓐ ⓑ ⓒ ⓓ
15. ⓐ ⓑ ⓒ ⓓ
16. ⓐ ⓑ ⓒ ⓓ
17. ⓐ ⓑ ⓒ ⓓ
18. ⓐ ⓑ ⓒ ⓓ
19. ⓐ ⓑ ⓒ ⓓ
20. ⓐ ⓑ ⓒ ⓓ
21. ⓐ ⓑ ⓒ ⓓ
22. ⓐ ⓑ ⓒ ⓓ
23. ⓐ ⓑ ⓒ ⓓ
24. ⓐ ⓑ ⓒ ⓓ
25. ⓐ ⓑ ⓒ ⓓ
26. ⓐ ⓑ ⓒ ⓓ
27. ⓐ ⓑ ⓒ ⓓ
28. ⓐ ⓑ ⓒ ⓓ
29. ⓐ ⓑ ⓒ ⓓ
30. ⓐ ⓑ ⓒ ⓓ
31. ⓐ ⓑ ⓒ ⓓ
32. ⓐ ⓑ ⓒ ⓓ
33. ⓐ ⓑ ⓒ ⓓ
34. ⓐ ⓑ ⓒ ⓓ
35. ⓐ ⓑ ⓒ ⓓ
36. ⓐ ⓑ ⓒ ⓓ
37. ⓐ ⓑ ⓒ ⓓ
38. ⓐ ⓑ ⓒ ⓓ
39. ⓐ ⓑ ⓒ ⓓ
40. ⓐ ⓑ ⓒ ⓓ
41. ⓐ ⓑ ⓒ ⓓ
42. ⓐ ⓑ ⓒ ⓓ
43. ⓐ ⓑ ⓒ ⓓ
44. ⓐ ⓑ ⓒ ⓓ
45. ⓐ ⓑ ⓒ ⓓ
46. ⓐ ⓑ ⓒ ⓓ
47. ⓐ ⓑ ⓒ ⓓ
48. ⓐ ⓑ ⓒ ⓓ
49. ⓐ ⓑ ⓒ ⓓ
50. ⓐ ⓑ ⓒ ⓓ
51. ⓐ ⓑ ⓒ ⓓ
52. ⓐ ⓑ ⓒ ⓓ
53. ⓐ ⓑ ⓒ ⓓ
54. ⓐ ⓑ ⓒ ⓓ
55. ⓐ ⓑ ⓒ ⓓ
56. ⓐ ⓑ ⓒ ⓓ
57. ⓐ ⓑ ⓒ ⓓ
58. ⓐ ⓑ ⓒ ⓓ
59. ⓐ ⓑ ⓒ ⓓ
60. ⓐ ⓑ ⓒ ⓓ
61. ⓐ ⓑ ⓒ ⓓ
62. ⓐ ⓑ ⓒ ⓓ
63. ⓐ ⓑ ⓒ ⓓ
64. ⓐ ⓑ ⓒ ⓓ
65. ⓐ ⓑ ⓒ ⓓ
66. ⓐ ⓑ ⓒ ⓓ
67. ⓐ ⓑ ⓒ ⓓ
68. ⓐ ⓑ ⓒ ⓓ
69. ⓐ ⓑ ⓒ ⓓ
70. ⓐ ⓑ ⓒ ⓓ
71. ⓐ ⓑ ⓒ ⓓ
72. ⓐ ⓑ ⓒ ⓓ
73. ⓐ ⓑ ⓒ ⓓ
74. ⓐ ⓑ ⓒ ⓓ
75. ⓐ ⓑ ⓒ ⓓ
76. ⓐ ⓑ ⓒ ⓓ
77. ⓐ ⓑ ⓒ ⓓ
78. ⓐ ⓑ ⓒ ⓓ
79. ⓐ ⓑ ⓒ ⓓ
80. ⓐ ⓑ ⓒ ⓓ
81. ⓐ ⓑ ⓒ ⓓ
82. ⓐ ⓑ ⓒ ⓓ
83. ⓐ ⓑ ⓒ ⓓ
84. ⓐ ⓑ ⓒ ⓓ
85. ⓐ ⓑ ⓒ ⓓ
86. ⓐ ⓑ ⓒ ⓓ
87. ⓐ ⓑ ⓒ ⓓ
88. ⓐ ⓑ ⓒ ⓓ
89. ⓐ ⓑ ⓒ ⓓ
90. ⓐ ⓑ ⓒ ⓓ
91. ⓐ ⓑ ⓒ ⓓ
92. ⓐ ⓑ ⓒ ⓓ
93. ⓐ ⓑ ⓒ ⓓ
94. ⓐ ⓑ ⓒ ⓓ
95. ⓐ ⓑ ⓒ ⓓ
96. ⓐ ⓑ ⓒ ⓓ
97. ⓐ ⓑ ⓒ ⓓ
98. ⓐ ⓑ ⓒ ⓓ
99. ⓐ ⓑ ⓒ ⓓ
100. ⓐ ⓑ ⓒ ⓓ
101. ⓐ ⓑ ⓒ ⓓ
102. ⓐ ⓑ ⓒ ⓓ
103. ⓐ ⓑ ⓒ ⓓ
104. ⓐ ⓑ ⓒ ⓓ
105. ⓐ ⓑ ⓒ ⓓ
106. ⓐ ⓑ ⓒ ⓓ
107. ⓐ ⓑ ⓒ ⓓ
108. ⓐ ⓑ ⓒ ⓓ
109. ⓐ ⓑ ⓒ ⓓ
110. ⓐ ⓑ ⓒ ⓓ
111. ⓐ ⓑ ⓒ ⓓ
112. ⓐ ⓑ ⓒ ⓓ
113. ⓐ ⓑ ⓒ ⓓ
114. ⓐ ⓑ ⓒ ⓓ
115. ⓐ ⓑ ⓒ ⓓ
116. ⓐ ⓑ ⓒ ⓓ
117. ⓐ ⓑ ⓒ ⓓ
118. ⓐ ⓑ ⓒ ⓓ
119. ⓐ ⓑ ⓒ ⓓ
120. ⓐ ⓑ ⓒ ⓓ
121. ⓐ ⓑ ⓒ ⓓ
122. ⓐ ⓑ ⓒ ⓓ
123. ⓐ ⓑ ⓒ ⓓ
124. ⓐ ⓑ ⓒ ⓓ
125. ⓐ ⓑ ⓒ ⓓ
126. ⓐ ⓑ ⓒ ⓓ
127. ⓐ ⓑ ⓒ ⓓ
128. ⓐ ⓑ ⓒ ⓓ
129. ⓐ ⓑ ⓒ ⓓ
130. ⓐ ⓑ ⓒ ⓓ
131. ⓐ ⓑ ⓒ ⓓ
132. ⓐ ⓑ ⓒ ⓓ
133. ⓐ ⓑ ⓒ ⓓ
134. ⓐ ⓑ ⓒ ⓓ
135. ⓐ ⓑ ⓒ ⓓ
136. ⓐ ⓑ ⓒ ⓓ
137. ⓐ ⓑ ⓒ ⓓ
138. ⓐ ⓑ ⓒ ⓓ
139. ⓐ ⓑ ⓒ ⓓ
140. ⓐ ⓑ ⓒ ⓓ
141. ⓐ ⓑ ⓒ ⓓ
142. ⓐ ⓑ ⓒ ⓓ
143. ⓐ ⓑ ⓒ ⓓ
144. ⓐ ⓑ ⓒ ⓓ
145. ⓐ ⓑ ⓒ ⓓ
146. ⓐ ⓑ ⓒ ⓓ
147. ⓐ ⓑ ⓒ ⓓ
148. ⓐ ⓑ ⓒ ⓓ
149. ⓐ ⓑ ⓒ ⓓ
150. ⓐ ⓑ ⓒ ⓓ
151. ⓐ ⓑ ⓒ ⓓ
152. ⓐ ⓑ ⓒ ⓓ
153. ⓐ ⓑ ⓒ ⓓ
154. ⓐ ⓑ ⓒ ⓓ
155. ⓐ ⓑ ⓒ ⓓ
156. ⓐ ⓑ ⓒ ⓓ
157. ⓐ ⓑ ⓒ ⓓ
158. ⓐ ⓑ ⓒ ⓓ
159. ⓐ ⓑ ⓒ ⓓ
160. ⓐ ⓑ ⓒ ⓓ
161. ⓐ ⓑ ⓒ ⓓ
162. ⓐ ⓑ ⓒ ⓓ
163. ⓐ ⓑ ⓒ ⓓ
164. ⓐ ⓑ ⓒ ⓓ
165. ⓐ ⓑ ⓒ ⓓ

Questions

1. The nurse on a medical-surgical unit is caring for a client with an extensive wound infection. The physician has ordered contact precautions based on the wound culture results. The nurse recognizes when caring for this client that she should wear disposable medical examination gloves

a. upon entering the client's room to provide care.
b. when providing care within five feet of the client.
c. when anticipating a dressing change.
d. when the potential of contamination from body fluids exists.

2. When administering magnesium to a pre-eclampsic pregnant woman, the nurse assesses for signs and symptoms of magnesium toxicity. These include all of the following EXCEPT

a. absent reflexes.
b. fetal heart rate of 120.
c. respirations < 12 per minute.
d. urine output < 30cc/hour.

3. The nurse is caring for a client diagnosed with glaucoma. Which of the following medications, if prescribed for the client, should the nurse question?

a. atropine sulfate (Isopto Atropine)
b. betaxolol (Betoptic)
c. pilocarpine (Ocusert Pilo-20)
d. pilocarpine hydrochloride (Isopto Carpine)

4. Upon examining the mouth and throat of a seven-year-old, the nurse observes the following:

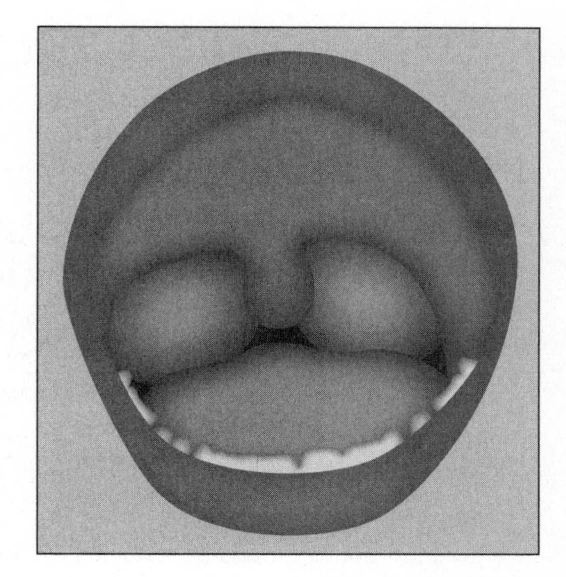

The mother asks the nurse if the child's tonsils should be removed as they are so large. The nurse knows that the tonsils reach their maximum size between the ages of

a. 4 and 6.
b. 6 and 8.
c. 8 and 10.
d. 10 and 12.

5. The nurse is preparing to complete a neurological assessment on a client. The nurse is aware that which of the following are included when assessing a client using the Glasgow Coma Scale? Select all that apply.

1. eye opening
2. motor response
3. pupil reaction
4. verbal performance

a. 1, 2, 3, 4
b. 1, 2, 4
c. 1, 4
d. 2, 3

6. When the nurse is able to take the client's perspective into consideration and communicate this understanding back to the client, the nurse is using

a. assertiveness.
b. empathy.
c. sympathy.
d. transference.

7. A nurse administers 12 U of regular insulin mixed with 34 U of NPH insulin to a diabetic client at 7:00 a.m. At 12 noon the client is off the unit at radiology when lunch trays arrive. Which of the following is the most appropriate action for the nurse to complete?

a. Contact the radiology department and ask the RN to start an IV of 5% dextrose.
b. Request that the client be returned to the unit to eat lunch if the testing is not complete.
c. Save the lunch tray and have client eat when he or she returns to the unit.
d. Take a glass of orange juice or milk to the radiology department for the client at 12 noon.

8. A woman in preterm labor is admitted to the hospital and given an intramuscular (IM) injection of betamethasone. The nurse explains to the client that betamethasone

a. lowers maternal blood pressure.
b. prevents fetal seizures.
c. promotes fetal lung maturation.
d. stops maternal contractions.

9. A nurse has asked an unlicensed nursing assistant to feed a client who is ordered a full liquid diet. The nurse will instruct the nursing assistant that which of the following items are permitted on this type of diet? Select all that apply.

1. ice cream
2. oatmeal
3. pudding
4. yogurt

a. 1, 4
b. 2, 3
c. 1, 3, 4
d. 1, 2, 4

10. The nurse is teaching a class to new mothers about safe infant sleeping environments. The nurse teaches that which of the following increase the infant's risk for sudden infant death syndrome (SIDS)? Select all that apply.

1. sleeping with a pacifier
2. low birth weight
3. maternal smoking during pregnancy
4. being placed on back for sleep

a. 1, 2
b. 2, 3
c. 3, 4
d. 1, 4

11. The nurse is caring for a client in the intensive, care unit (ICU) who has suffered a stroke. The client is diagnosed with a left homonymous hemianopsia. Which of the following illustrations demonstrates the nurse's interpretation of the visual field defect that this client is experiencing?

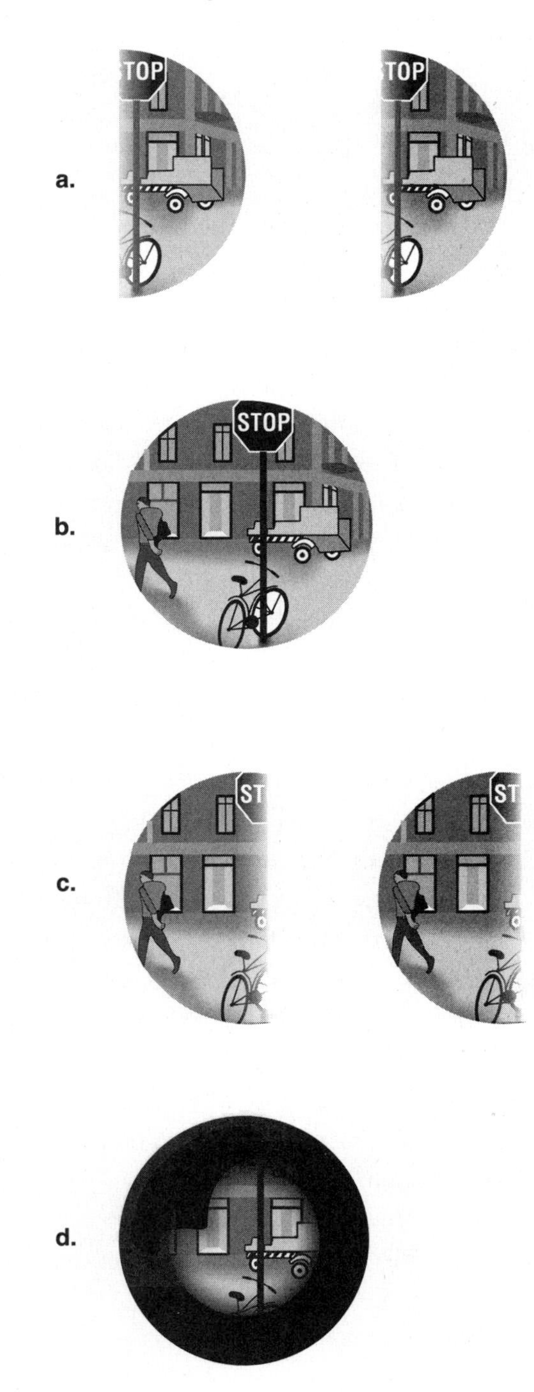

12. The first intervention that a nurse should perform when caring for a woman experiencing postpartum hemorrhage due to uterine atony is to
a. administer packed red blood cells.
b. administer pitocin.
c. insert a urinary catheter.
d. massage the fundus.

13. A client on a medical surgical unit is extremely restless and agitated. It is decided that the client will begin chemical restraints with IV sedatives. The nurse recognizes it is important to monitor the client for which of the following common side effects associated with chemical sedations and restraints?
a. ability to remove the restraints
b. pain
c. hypertension
d. respiratory depression

14. A nurse goes into a client's room to start an IV. The client tells the nurse in a hostile voice, "I am sick of being poked at and stuck with needles. Go away and leave me alone." Which is the best response by the nurse?
a. "I will leave you alone."
b. "This won't hurt."
c. "You have had a lot of tests and treatments."
d. "You have to have this IV."

15. A client is being prepared for cardioversion. The client is fearful and anxious about the pain associated with the countershock to be delivered. Conscious sedation is provided for the client. The nurse will monitor the client for which of the following associated with conscious sedation?
a. allergic reaction
b. alteration in level of consciousness
c. hypertension
d. respiratory distress

16. The nurse is working with a client on the one-year anniversary of a stillborn baby's birth. The client expresses that for the past month she has been experiencing episodes of sadness and crying. The nurse knows that most likely this client is in which of the following phases of grief?

a. anticipatory
b. bittersweet
c. intense
d. reorganization

17. A client with positive cultures for methicillin-resistant Staphylococcus aureus (MRSA) is being treated on a medical-surgical unit. The nurses on the unit implement contact precautions when interacting with the client. Which of the following are components of contact precautions?

a. placing the client in a negative air pressure room
b. placing the client in a private or semiprivate room
c. wearing an N-95 respirator when interacting with the client
d. wearing a mask when interacting with the client

18. The nurse is assessing a six-month-old with hydrocephalus. The nurse would expect to find which of the following upon assessment?

a. bulging fontanel
b. firm fontanel
c. increased pulse
d. sunken fontanel

19. The nurse is assisting a client to the bathroom. During the interaction, the client tells the nurse, "I might as well be dead; I can't even go to the bathroom on my own." Which response by the nurse would be most therapeutic and appropriate?

a. "Stay positive. Things will look better tomorrow."
b. "You are progressing well. A week ago, you couldn't even get out of bed."
c. "You sound really discouraged and frustrated today."
d. "Why are you feeling so bad today? This isn't like you."

20. The nurse is trying to teach an eight-year-old girl how to administer her insulin injections. The girl is accompanied by her mother and her sister, who is a toddler. The toddler keeps interrupting the nurse. What strategy might the nurse use to facilitate communication?

a. Distract the toddler with a book.
b. Ignore the toddler and continue.
c. Tell the toddler to behave.
d. Tell the mother to control the toddler.

21. The nurse is caring for a client diagnosed with Alzheimer's who is being treated for pneumonia. During a.m. care, the client becomes agitated and states, "Where am I? I'm afraid. Who are you? Where is my family?" Which of the following is the nurse's best response?

a. "I just told you four times that you're in the hospital and your family will be here later."
b. "The name of the hospital is on the sign over the door. Let's go out into the hall and read it again."
c. "You are in the hospital and you're safe. Your family will be here at 10 o'clock, which is half an hour from now."
d. "You know where you are. You were admitted here one week ago for pneumonia. Don't worry; your family will be here soon."

22. The nurse anticipates administering methotrexate for which of the following complications in the antepartum period?
a. complete abortion
b. ruptured tubal pregnancy
c. threatened abortion
d. unruptured tubal pregnancy

23. The nurse is caring for a client with a Pleur-Evac chest tube following open heart surgery. On the illustration, which area should the nurse check when assessing for the presence of an air leak?

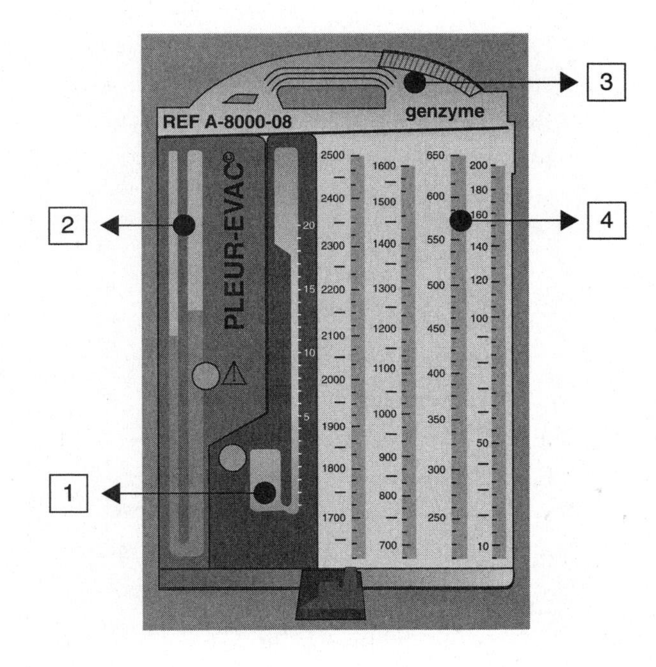

a. 1
b. 2
c. 3
d. 4

24. A nurse working in a child development clinic notices that a child consistently plays alone, even when other children are present. While the child enjoys the presence of others, she focuses on her own activity. The nurse recognizes that solitary play is appropriate for which age child?
a. an infant
b. a toddler
c. a preschooler
d. a school age child

25. The nurse identifies a client as being at risk for developing thromboembolic disease. Antiembolism stockings have been ordered for the client. Which of the following directions should the nurse include in teaching the client about the correct use of the stockings?
a. If ambulating at least 10 times daily, it is unnecessary to wear the stockings.
b. If the skin becomes painful underneath the stockings, notify the nurse and request pain medication.
c. Cross the legs only while wearing the stockings; otherwise keep the legs uncrossed.
d. The most appropriate time to apply the hose is before standing first thing in the morning.

26. A woman comes into the office for her initial prenatal visit. She states the first day of her last menstrual period was April 9, 2012. Using Naegele's rule, the nurse determines the client's correct due date to be
a. January 9, 2013
b. January 16, 2013
c. January 23, 2013
d. January 26, 2013

27. A client has undergone emergency treatment related to acute coronary syndrome. The client has had minimal periods of sleep over the past 24 hours. Which of the following assessment findings is consistent with sleep deprivation?
a. cool extremities
b. confusion
c. depression
d. periods of apnea

28. The nurse has been asked by the manager to work an overtime shift. She does not want the overtime because of an evening appointment. The manager tells her to think of her coworkers, who will have a "bad" evening if the "hole" is not filled. The best assertive response from the nurse is,
a. "I cannot work the shift tonight."
b. "Okay, I will this time but not the next."
c. "You are making me feel guilty."
d. "You don't understand."

29. The nurse is completing her morning assessment on her assigned client. The nurse notes that the client's blood pressure is 85/55 mm Hg with a pulse rate of 62 bpm. Which of the following actions should the nurse complete first?
a. Assess the client for dizziness and the skin of the extremities for warmth.
b. Elevate the head of the client's bed.
c. Retake the client's blood pressure.
d. Review the client's chart and determine the client's normal blood pressure range.

30. The nurse is teaching the parent of a child with eczema (atopic dermatitis). The nurse determines that the parent understands the instructions when the parent states that when bathing the child she will
a. ensure the child's skin is completely dry after bathing.
b. use a mild soap or cleansing agent.
c. use hot water.
d. vigorously rub the child with a towel.

31. The nurse is caring for a client who is hyperthermic. The physician orders the application of a hypothermic blanket. Which of the following findings should lead the nurse to suspect the client may be experiencing hypothermia following the application of the blanket? Select all that apply.
1. bradycardia
2. drowsiness
3. hypertension
4. hypotension
5. increased urine output
6. tachycardia

a. 1, 2, 4
b. 2, 4, 5
c. 2, 3, 6
d. 3, 5, 6

32. A laboring client's station is documented as −1. The nurse assuming care for this client would expect the fetal head to be
a. crowning.
b. level with the ischial spines.
c. one centimeter above the ischial spines.
d. one centimeter below the ischial spines.

33. A nurse is assessing the pupil size of a client diagnosed with an epidural hematoma. Following the assessment, the nurse immediately notifies the physician that the client may be experiencing increased intracranial pressure with compression of the oculomotor nerve. Which of the following pupil sizes on the illustration best supports the nurse's conclusion?

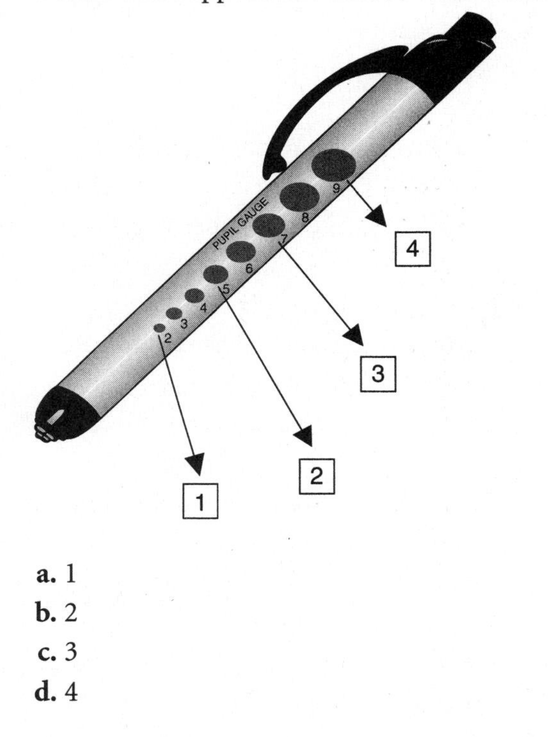

a. 1
b. 2
c. 3
d. 4

34. A 13-year-old enters a hospital for a surgical procedure. The nurse planning care for the adolescent knows that
a. development ends in adolescence.
b. growth is proximocaudal.
c. growth is cephalodistal.
d. developmental tasks are age-related.

35. A seasoned nurse is passing medications with a graduate nurse. The graduate nurse is preparing to apply a clonidine (Catapres) transdermal patch to a client. Which of the following actions by the graduate nurse would cause the seasoned nurse to intervene?
a. The graduate nurse applies a bioclusive seal over the patch after application.
b. The graduate nurse applies the patch to a dry, hairless area of subcutaneous tissue.
c. The graduate nurse performs hand hygiene after the application of the patch.
d. The graduate nurse removes any previously applied transdermal patch.

36. The nurse is caring for a postpartum woman experiencing hemorrhagic shock. The nurse recognizes that the most objective and least invasive assessment of adequate organ perfusion and oxygenation is
a. cool, dry skin.
b. cyanosis in the buccal mucosa.
c. diminished restlessness.
d. urinary output at least 30 ml/hour.

37. The nurse is preparing to administer an intramuscular (IM) injection into the left dorsogluteal muscle of an adult client. On the illustration, in which area should the nurse plan to administer the injection?

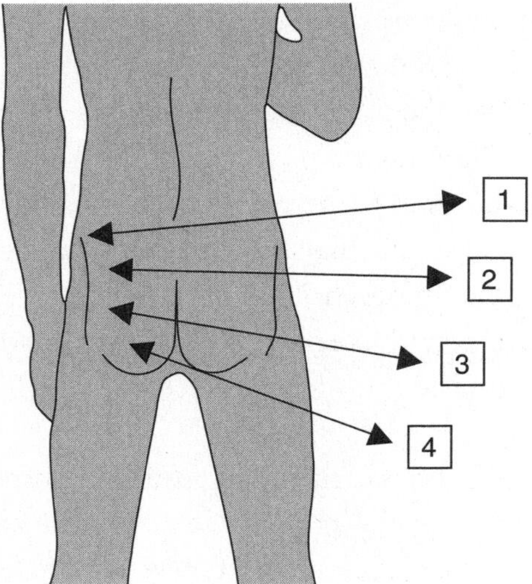

a. 1
b. 2
c. 3
d. 4

38. The nurse has just completed reading a client's biopsy report, which shows that the client has cancer. As the nurse enters the room to perform an assessment, the client states: "I know that the biopsies will show I have cancer." The nurse's best response is,
a. "I do not know what the biopsies will show."
b. "I am not allowed to discuss the results."
c. "Maybe you don't have cancer."
d. "You think the biopsies will be positive?"

39. The nurse is caring for a client who is receiving IV gentamicin. The nurse recognizes that gentamicin is known to be nephrotoxic. Given these circumstances, the nurse should independently evaluate the client's
a. BUN level.
b. creatinine clearance level.
c. fluid intake.
d. urinary output.

40. A six-year-old boy is being seen at an urgent-care clinic. Upon assessing the respiratory rate, the nurse determines it to be 24 breaths per minute. The most appropriate action by the nurse is to
a. document the respiratory rate.
b. have another nurse recheck the rate.
c. notify the physician.
d. recheck the respiratory rate.

41. The nurse is caring for a client diagnosed with cirrhosis. Which of the following information obtained by the nurse during the assessment will be of most concern?
a. The client has ascites and a 3 kg weight gain from the previous day.
b. The client complains of right upper-quadrant pain with abdominal palpation.
c. The client's skin has multiple spider-shaped blood vessels on the abdomen.
d. The client's hands flap back and forth when the arms are extended.

42. When assessing for fetal presentation on a pregnant client, the nurse should use which of the following?
a. Chadwick's sign
b. Hegar's sign
c. Leopold's maneuver
d. McMurray's test

43. The nurse is working with a dying client who states that he told God that if he could just live to see his son's graduation, he could die in peace. The nurse should document that the client is in which of the following stages of death and dying, according to Dr. Elisabeth Kübler-Ross's theories?

a. anger
b. bargaining
c. denial
d. depression

44. A client on a medical-surgical unit diagnosed with hypertension is receiving the diuretic spironolactone (Aldactone). Which of the following statements by the client indicates that the teaching about this medication has been effective?

a. "I can only have low-fat cheese."
b. "I can use a salt substitute at dinner."
c. "I will have apple juice instead of orange juice."
d. "I will drink at least six glasses of water every day."

45. The nurse is preparing to care for a pregnant client whose medical record documents that the client has +1 protein in her urine and a blood pressure reading of 152/92. The nurse plans care for a client most likely experiencing

a. eclampsia.
b. gestational hypertension.
c. preeclampsia.
d. severe preeclampsia.

46. A 56-year-old female client asks the nurse how to calculate her body mass index (BMI). The client weighs 160 pounds and is 5 feet 6 inches tall (66″). Together, the client and the nurse calculate the client's BMI to the nearest tenth of a point as which of the following?

a. 25.8
b. 24.7
c. 24.9
d. 23.9

47. The nurse is conducting a parenting class for new parents. The nurse correctly instructs the parents that infant social development includes smiling at their mirror image during which of the following ages?

a. zero to three months
b. four to six months
c. seven to nine months
d. 10 to 12 months

48. The nurse is caring for a client with a stage 3 pressure ulcer. The client's daughter asks the nurse which layer of her mother's tissue is actually damaged. Using the illustration, the nurse indicates which circled area is indicative of a stage 3 pressure ulcer?

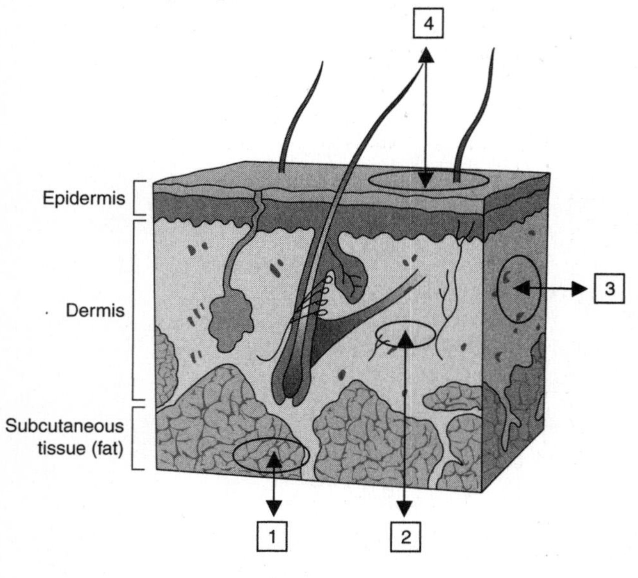

a. 1
b. 2
c. 3
d. 4

49. The nurse makes a phone call to the physician regarding a 79-year-old client with chest pains. The client has a history of anxiety. The nurse correctly communicates the information indicated in the "B" of the SBAR communication technique in which of the following statements?
a. "A 79-year-old client with a history of anxiety."
b. "He is complaining of chest pain."
c. "Do you want to start an EKG?"
d. "I am concerned about a panic attack."

50. The nurse is completing an admission assessment on a client who is having a same-day procedure. The client states she has been taking ginkgo daily for the past year. To monitor the effectiveness of ginkgo, the nurse evaluates which of the following?
a. blood pressure
b. motivation
c. attention span
d. red blood cells

51. When assessing the cervix of a client thought to be about four weeks pregnant, the nurse determines that the lower portion of the client's cervix is beginning to soften. The nurse should document this as
a. Chadwick's sign.
b. Hegar's sign.
c. Homan's sign.
d. Murphy's sign.

52. A client diagnosed with terminal brain cancer is admitted into a hospice program. The client is experiencing continuous, increasing amounts of pain. The nurse caring for the client will administer opioid pain medications to provide which of the following?
a. around-the-clock routine administration of analgesics
b. enough pain medication to keep the client comfortable
c. pain relief with *pro re nata* (PRN) medications at the client's request
d. sedation and pain relief at the family's request

53. The nurse is assessing the skin of a six-year-old boy with severe cerebral palsy and notes that the child has a pressure ulcer on the right buttock measuring 2 cm by 2 cm with partial-thickness loss of the dermis. She also observes that the wound base is red. The nurse should document this pressure ulcer as
a. stage 1.
b. stage 2.
c. stage 3.
d. stage 4.

54. A client arrives in the emergency department with a swollen right ankle after an injury while playing football. Which of the following initial actions by the nurse is most appropriate?
a. appling a moist, warm compress to the ankle.
b. assessing ROM of the right ankle
c. removing the client's cleat and sock
d. wrapping the ankle in a compression bandage

55. The nurse is assessing a newborn infant. Which of the following is a sign of potential distress?
a. closed posterior fontanel
b. heart rate of 130
c. palpable anterior fontanel
d. respiratory rate of 40

56. The nurse enters the room of a client who has just returned from surgery. The client had a total laryngectomy and radical neck dissection. Upon assessment, the nurse notes the following problems. In which order should the nurse address them?
1. The client is coughing blood-tinged secretions from the tracheostomy.
2. The client is lying in a lateral position with the head of the bed flat.
3. The Hemovac in the neck incision contains 250 mL of bloody drainage.
4. The NG tube is disconnected from suction and clamped off.

a. 1, 2, 3, 4
b. 2, 1, 3, 4
c. 4, 2, 1, 3
d. 4, 3, 2, 1

57. The nurse is working with a client who has depression. The client exhibits some signs of regressing and mourning over an impending loss but demonstrates satisfaction and competence. The nurse and client are in which phase of the therapeutic relationship?
a. initiating
b. orienting
c. termination
d. working

58. The nurse is caring for a client receiving chemotherapy. Which of the following laboratory results is most important to report to the healthcare provider?
a. hemoglobin of 11 g/L
b. platelets of 66,000/μl
c. serum creatinine level of 1.0 mg/dl
d. WBC count of 1,800/μl

59. A nurse at an urgent-care clinic is assessing a 13-month-old child with diarrhea. The nurse checks for signs of dehydration by assessing the child for a

a. bulging fontanel.
b. closed fontanel.
c. firm fontanel.
d. sunken fontanel.

60. A bone marrow transplant is being planned for a client with acute leukemia who has not responded to chemotherapy. In discussing this treatment with the client, the nurse will explain which of the following?

a. The donor bone marrow cells are transplanted immediately after an infusion of chemotherapy.
b. The transplantation of the donated cells is considered painful by many clients.
c. The transplant procedure takes place in a sterile operating room to minimize the risk for infection.
d. Several weeks of hospitalization will be required after the hematopoietic stem cell transplant (HSCT).

61. The nurse is determining a neonate's Apgar score one minute after birth. The neonate's central skin color is pink but all extremities are blue. The nurse should score the infant's color as which of the following?

a. 0
b. 1
c. 2
d. 3

62. The nurse is developing a plan of care for a client diagnosed with syndrome of inappropriate antidiuretic hormone (SIADH). Which of the following interventions would be most important for the nurse to include in the care of this client?

a. ambulating the client once a shift
b. instructing the client to use incentive spirometry every two hours
c. monitoring hourly intake and output
d. restricting free water oral intake

63. The nurse is admitting a male client with borderline personality disorder. When conducting the client's health history, the nurse would NOT expect to find which of the following?

a. impulsive behavior
b. persistent mistrust of others
c. low self-esteem
d. substance abuse

64. A client in the ICU is ordered to receive IV potassium chloride (KCL) 40 mEq for the treatment of hypokalemia. When administering the potassium solution via a central line, the nurse is aware that which of the following is true?

a. The amount of KCL added to IV fluids should not exceed 20 mEq/L to prevent the development of hyperkalemia.
b. The KCL should be administered as an IV bolus in order to correct the hypokalemia quickly before complications occur.
c. The KCL should be given very slowly to avoid venospasm and inflammation at the IV insertion site.
d. To reduce the risk for cardiac dysrhythmia, the maximum amount of KCL to be administered in one hour should not exceed 20 mEq.

65. The nurse begins the assessment process of a child during a well-baby visit. The nurse notices the infant using the pincer grasp to pick up pieces of cereal and eat them unassisted. Based on the infant's fine motor development, the nurse should recognize an infant who is approximately how many months old?
a. one
b. four
c. eight
d. 11

66. A client has undergone a cataract extraction and intraocular lens implantation. On the third postoperative day the client contacts the eye clinic and gives the nurse all of the following information. Which information is most concerning to the nurse?
a. The client complains that the vision has "not improved much."
b. The client complains of eye pain rated at a 6 (on a 0–10 scale).
c. The client has poor depth perception when wearing the eye patch.
d. The client has questions about the prescribed eyedrops.

67. The nurse is assessing the head and chest circumference of a one-week-old infant. The nurse expects the head circumference to be
a. larger than the chest by 2–3 cm.
b. larger than the chest by 4–5 cm.
c. smaller than the chest by 2–3 cm.
d. smaller than the chest by 4–5 cm.

68. A client with Ménière's disease is admitted to the hospital with vertigo, nausea, and vomiting. Which of the following nursing interventions is appropriate for the nurse to implement?
a. Encourage oral fluids up to 2,000 mL daily.
b. Change the client's position every four hours.
c. Keep the head of the bed elevated at 30 degrees.
d. Keep the client's room darkened and quiet.

69. The nurse working with preadolescent and adolescent girls knows that females should receive three doses of the HPV vaccine, according to Centers for Disease Control and Prevention (CDC) recommendations, between the ages of
a. 7 and 9.
b. 10 and 12.
c. 13 and 18.
d. 18 and 21.

70. A client is brought to the trauma center by a coworker after suffering a burn injury while working on an electrical power line. Which of the following actions should the nurse complete first?
a. Assess for the contact points.
b. Obtain the client's vital signs.
c. Place a cervical collar on the client.
d. Place the client on a cardiac monitor.

71. The nurse is caring for a client with a history of drinking a case of beer per day. The client underwent an emergency appendectomy. Knowing that the client is at risk for withdrawal symptoms, the nurse's plan of care includes an assessment for all of the following EXCEPT
a. agitation.
b. decreased heart rate.
c. hyperalertness.
d. seizures.

72. A male client diagnosed with sleep apnea has been using a Continuous Positive Airway Pressure (CPAP) machine for two weeks. When the client returns to the sleep clinic, he tells the nurse, "I still am not sleeping well." Which of the following responses by the nurse is most appropriate?

a. "CPAP takes a month or so to achieve the maximum effect."
b. "Do you want to talk to the physician about possible surgery?"
c. "Have you been using the CPAP every night as instructed?"
d. "It is possible the CPAP pressure should be increased."

73. A nurse is precepting a nursing student who is caring for a pregnant client with a low-lying placenta previa. The nurse determines that the student is able to differentiate between the types of placenta previa when the student identifies which of the following as a low-lying placenta previa?

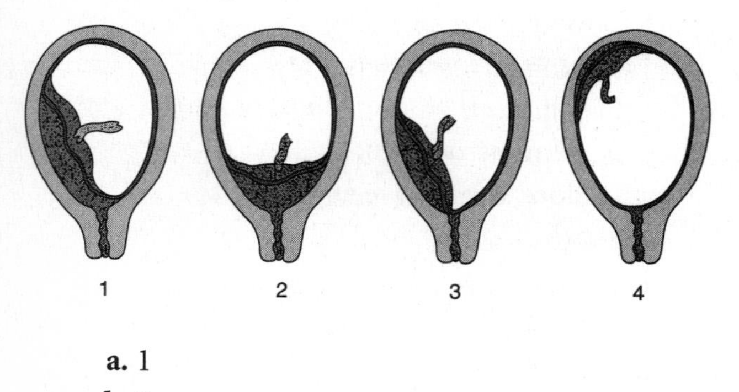

a. 1
b. 2
c. 3
d. 4

74. The nurse is reviewing orders written by the physician after making client rounds. After reviewing the orders, the nurse determines which of the following require the nurse to contact the physician to clarify the order? Select all that apply.

1. aspirin 325 mg orally qd
2. furosemide (Lasix) 20 mg IV now
3. D5W with 40 mEq KCL IV at 150 mL/hr.
4. heparin 5,000 u subcutaneously b.id.
5. MS 2 mg IV q 1hr PRN

a. 1, 2, 3, 4
b. 1, 4, 5
c. 2, 3, 5
d. 1, 2

75. A nurse is working at the emergency department when a young child is admitted with poisoning. The nurse suspects that the poisoning agent was a corrosive substance when which of the following is assessed?

a. drooling
b. jaundice
c. oliguria
d. tinnitus

76. The nurse is assessing a female client after surgery. The client states that she has been utilizing aromatherapy. The nurse will evaluate the effects of aromatherapy on the client by completing which of the following?

a. auscultating the client's breath sounds
b. assessing the client's blood pressure and heart rate
c. checking the incision for signs of infection
d. monitoring the client's intake and output

77. A client in labor has the following fetal heart monitor tracing:

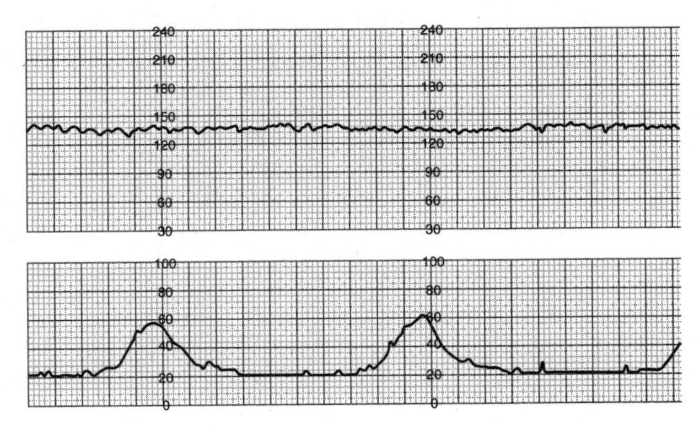

Which intervention should the nurse implement first?

a. Continue to monitor client.
b. Notify the physician.
c. Place client in left lateral position.
d. Prepare for an emergency cesarean section.

78. A client who is recovering from orthopedic surgery is seen in the clinic two weeks later. The client has been instructed to use a walker to ambulate with partial weight bearing. Which of the following observations would lead the nurse to conclude the client is using the correct technique?

a. The client's elbows are bent at a 30° angle while using the walker.
b. The client is bent over the walker.
c. The client holds the walker about two inches above the floor while walking.
d. The client is utilizing a walker that has four wheels in place.

79. A client is admitted into the emergency room with a suspected cocaine overdose. The nurse knows that this client is at risk for

a. cardiac arrest.
b. panic.
c. psychosis.
d. respiratory arrest.

80. The nurse has administered lactulose (Cephulac) 30 mL QID over the course of the hospitalization of a client diagnosed with advanced cirrhosis. The client is now complaining of diarrhea. The nurse explains to the client that it is still important to take the lactulose because it

a. prevents constipation.
b. prevents gastrointestinal bleeding.
c. improves nervous system function.
d. promotes fluid loss.

81. A child is admitted to the acute-care facility due to pyloric stenosis. The nurse's plan of care should include all EXCEPT which of the following?

1. assessment for dehydration
2. administration of blood products
3. administration of chelation therapy
4. document intake and output

a. 1 and 2
b. 1 and 3
c. 2 and 3
d. 1 and 4

82. A nurse is preparing to care for a client who had a lobectomy for the treatment of lung cancer. Which of the following illustrations reflects the nurse's knowledge about the extent of surgery performed?

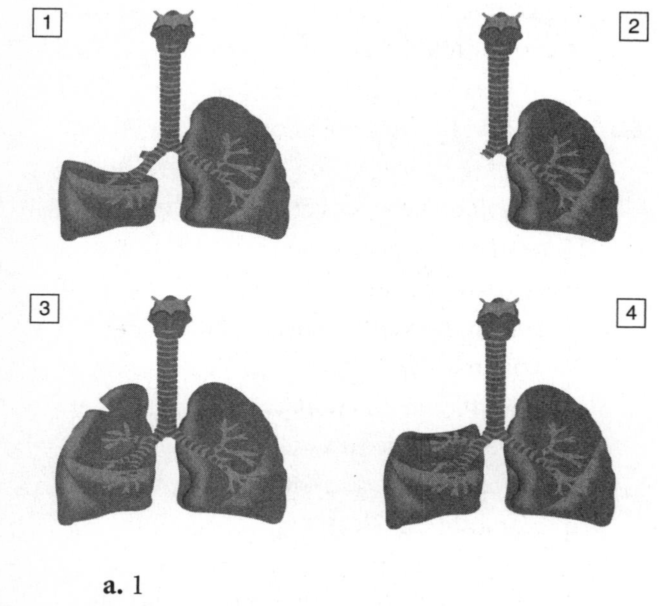

a. 1
b. 2
c. 3
d. 4

83. A nurse is providing nutritional education to a pregnant client. Which of the following foods should the nurse instruct the client to avoid?
a. hard-boiled eggs
b. morning cup of coffee
c. cooked shrimp
d. feta cheese

84. A nurse is inserting a nasogastric (NG) tube for a client diagnosed with a small bowel obstruction. While inserting the tube, resistance is met. Which of the following actions is most appropriate for the nurse to take next?
a. Ask the client to swallow some water.
b. Check for the correct placement of the tube with 30 cc of air.
c. Continue to advance or push the tube into the nares.
d. Remove the tube and try the other nares.

85. A client prescribed donepezil (Aricept) for treatment of Alzheimer's disease is being admitted into the hospital. During the review of medications, the nurse assesses for which class of medications that are contraindicated with Aricept?
a. anticholinergics
b. diuretics
c. narcotics
d. antipsychotics

86. A nurse is caring for a client who is receiving IV heparin after suffering a stroke. Which of the following laboratory results indicates that the client is receiving a therapeutic dosage?
a. phosphorus: 3.9 mg/dL
b. platelets: 275,000/mm^3
c. PT: 22 seconds
d. PTT: 60 seconds

87. The nurse is planning to provide education on safe infant sleeping practices to a new mother. The nurse realizes that the client will be most receptive to learning infant care during which of Rubin's phases of bonding?
a. letting-go phase
b. letting-in phase
c. taking-in phase
d. taking-hold phase

88. A nurse is caring for all of the following clients on a medical-surgical unit. Which of the following is at risk for developing respiratory acidosis?

a. a 30-year-old with Guillain-Barré syndrome
b. a 40-year-old with a large amount of pancreatic drainage
c. a 52-year-old who has received a massive blood transfusion
d. a 65-year-old with chronic congestive heart failure

89. The nurse is working on a neurologic pediatric unit. The nurse would suspect increased intercranial pressure in the child exhibiting which of the following symptoms?

a. decreased pulse and decreased blood pressure
b. decreased pulse and increased blood pressure
c. increased pulse and increased blood pressure
d. increased pulse and decreased blood pressure

90. A client had a splenectomy performed after experiencing a lacerated spleen from a motorcycle accident. The nurse will anticipate teaching the client about the increased risk for developing which of the following related to this surgical procedure?

a. anemia
b. bleeding tendencies
c. infection
d. lymphedema

91. A client has just delivered a newborn. The client begins to tremble as the placenta is delivered. The nurse recognizes that trembling

a. has no clinical significance.
b. indicates fear of becoming a mother.
c. indicates fear of fetal death.
d. indicates abruptio placentae.

92. An elderly female client with an extensive medical history is being treated in the CVICU for her third myocardial infarction. The client's family has encouraged her to complete a living will and a durable power of attorney. The client asks the nurse, "Why do I need to complete both?" The nurse explains to the client that a living will differs from a durable power of attorney in that the living will

a. authorizes a designated representative to act on the client's behalf in private affairs—medical, business, or some other legal matter.
b. provides a legal medical directive that specifies what types of medical treatment the client desires when or if she becomes unable to express her wishes.
c. provides the client with an advance health care directive (AHCD).
d. does not provide legal documentation of the client's wishes, but will make her family and healthcare providers quickly aware of her medical wishes.

93. A client has been prescribed Thorazine for relief of psychotic symptoms. The client later comes to the emergency room with symptoms of neuroleptic malignant syndrome. Upon assessment the nurse expects to find

a. dyskinesia.
b. gait shuffling.
c. rigidity.
d. toe tapping.

94. A client diagnosed with hypertensive crisis is admitted to the cardiac care unit (CCU). The client has no past medical history. Upon arrival to the unit, the client's blood pressure is 212/142 mm Hg. Which of the following findings during the nurse's reassessment will require immediate attention?
a. The client complains of a headache with a pain score of 8 on a scale of 1 to 10.
b. The client is unable to move the right leg when instructed.
c. The client's urine output is 85 mL over the past two hours.
d. Tremors are present in the fingers when the arms are extended.

95. A preceptor is working with a new nurse in the urgent-care clinic on the care of children with fevers. The preceptor determines that the new nurse has understood the related concepts when the new nurse instructs a mother NOT to give a child with a fever
a. acetaminophen.
b. acetylsalicylic acid.
c. ibuprofen.
d. tepid baths.

96. A client who weighs 155 pounds asks the nurse how much protein should be included in the daily diet. The nurse recommends that the diet should include which of the following minimums?
a. 38 grams of protein daily
b. 65 grams of protein daily
c. 53 grams of protein daily
d. 56 grams of protein daily

97. A client comes to the clinic due to suspected pregnancy. Upon sonographic exam, there is evidence of a fetus. The nurse knows this is a
a. positive sign of pregnancy.
b. potential sign of pregnancy.
c. presumptive sign of pregnancy.
d. probable sign of pregnancy.

98. A graduate nurse is caring for a client who is ordered soft wrist restraints. The graduate nurse asks the charge nurse how often she should plan to assess the placement of the restraints and the condition of the restrained area. Which of the following is the nurse's best response?
a. every half hour
b. every hour
c. every three hours
d. every eight hours

99. A client who is taking an antipsychotic is documented to have tardive dyskinesia. The nurse plans care for a client with
a. drooling, dystonia, and permanent gait shuffling.
b. pill-rolling movements, dyskinesia, and a flat affect.
c. spasms of the neck and limbs.
d. toe tapping and uncontrolled restlessness.

100. The nurse is caring for a client who is comatose following a head injury. The client is receiving continuous tube feedings via a soft nasogastric (NG) tube. During the nurse's reassessment of the client, new crackles in the client's lungs are noted. In which order will the nurse take the following actions?

1. Check the tube feeding residual volume.
2. Notify the client's physician.
3. Obtain the client's oxygen saturation.
4. Turn off the tube feeding.

a. 1, 3, 2, 4
b. 3, 1, 4, 2
c. 3, 4, 1, 2
d. 4, 3, 1, 2

101. The nurse is caring for a child admitted with acute glomerulonephritis. The nurse should incorporate which of the following into the plan of care?

a. decreased carbohydrates
b. decreased fluid
c. decreased protein
d. increased sodium

102. The nurse is caring for a client with an extensive burn injury. The nurse has calculated that the client needs 1,800 mL of fluid in the first 24 hours in order to maintain blood volume and urinary output. How many mL will the nurse plan to infuse in the first eight hours based on the Parkland formula?

a. 500
b. 700
c. 900
d. 1,200

103. The nurse is conducting a prenatal class and explaining cardinal movements of labor. The nurse determines that the class has understood the concepts when clients correctly identify the phase where the fetal head bends to the chest as

a. extension.
b. external rotation.
c. flexion.
d. internal rotation.

104. The nurse is caring for a client in the ICU with a central venous pressure (CVP) line. Which of the following is an appropriate practice guideline for the nurse to be aware of when CVP is being monitored?

a. A CVP of 2 to 5 mm Hg requires immediate intervention to prevent the development of pulmonary edema.
b. A CVP of 15 mm Hg or greater requires the need for immediate fluid replacement.
c. A pressure greater than 6 mm Hg must be reported to the physician immediately.
d. Overall trended measurements are more important than any individual measures.

105. A client's blood lithium level comes back as 0.9 mEq/L. The nurse's first intervention should be to

a. contact the physician with toxic level.
b. contact physician with therapeutic level.
c. continue to monitor the client.
d. prepare to administer mannitol.

106. A graduate nurse is following an RN during her nursing shift in the CCU. A client is to have an intra-arterial blood pressure monitoring initiated. The graduate nurse observes the nurse performing the Allen's test and asks why this test is completed. Which of the following is the best response by the nurse?

a. "To check for abnormal clotting because of the risk of thromboembolism formation.
b. "To check if the volume of blood flow is sufficient to the extremity to provide an accurate measurement."
c. "To determine if the artery has a diameter large enough to permit passage of the monitoring catheter."
d. "To make sure that collateral circulation is sufficient to keep the tissue supplied with oxygenated blood."

107. A laboring client's water breaks. The nurse suspects infection when the amniotic fluid is

a. clear with white flecks.
b. green in color.
c. port-wine color.
d. yellow.

108. The nurse is assessing a client experiencing the onset of symptoms of type 1 diabetes. Which of the following questions should the nurse ask the client?

a. "Do you crave sugary drinks?"
b. "Has your weight decreased?"
c. "How long have you felt anorexic?"
d. "Is your urine dark in color?"

109. The nurse is providing teaching to a breast-feeding mother of a 12-month-old infant with an egg, milk, wheat, and soy allergy. The nurse should explain that the allergens that can be transmitted through breast milk include which of the following? Select all that apply.

1. eggs
2. milk
3. wheat
4. soy

a. 1, 2, 4
b. 2, 3, 4
c. 1, 3, 4
d. all of the above

110. A client diagnosed with acute renal failure (ARF) has a serum potassium level of 6.5 mEq/L. The client is ordered IV glucose and insulin. Which of the following will the nurse evaluate to best determine the effectiveness of the medications?

a. blood glucose level
b. BUN and creatinine levels
c. electrocardiograph (ECG)
d. serum potassium level

111. The nurse is caring for a client experiencing delirium due to a metabolic imbalance. The nurse plans care for the client knowing that delirium

1. causes permanent impairment.
2. causes reversible cognitive deficits.
3. is precipitated by a defined event.
4. is self-limiting.

a. 1 and 3
b. 2 and 3
c. 2 and 4
d. 1 and 4

112. A client presents to the emergency department (ED) with a sudden onset of jaundice, nausea, and vomiting. Further assessment and laboratory results reveal hepatomegaly, abnormal liver function studies, and negative serologic testing for viral causes of hepatitis. Which of the following questions is most appropriate for the nurse to ask the client?

a. "Are you taking corticosteroids for any reason?"
b. "Do any of your family members have jaundice?"
c. "Do you use any over-the-counter medications?"
d. "Have you ever used IV drugs in the past?"

113. The nurse is helping a client prepare a birthing plan. The nurse explains that which of the following are risk factors that might indicate a need for a cesarean birth? Select all that apply.

1. placenta previa
2. anemia
3. genital herpes
4. puerpera

a. 1, 2
b. 2, 3
c. 2, 4
d. 1, 3

114. A client diagnosed with atrial fibrillation is receiving warfarin (Coumadin) 5 mg each day. The client's international normalized ratio (INR) is 1.8. Which of the following is the expected nursing action regarding changing the dosage of medication?

a. The INR level is too low. The warfarin dosage should be increased.
b. The INR level is too high. The warfarin dosage needs to be decreased.
c. The INR level is too high. The warfarin dosage needs to be increased.
d. The INR level is within the expected range. The warfarin dosage does not need to be adjusted.

115. The nurse is caring for a child admitted with a sickle-cell anemia sequestration crisis. The nurse plans care for a child with

a. decreased red blood cell production.
b. petechia and bruising.
c. pooling of blood in the spleen.
d. swollen hands and feet.

116. The nurse assesses a client's gag reflex. When doing so, which of the following cranial nerves is the nurse assessing?

a. Abducens (sixth)
b. Glossopharyngeal (ninth)
c. Hypoglossal (12th)
d. Trigeminal (fifth).

117. When timing a client's contractions, the nurse measures the frequency of the contractions by measuring from

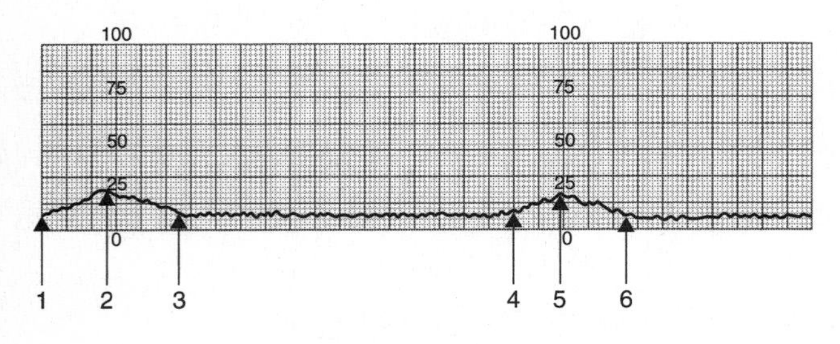

a. point 1 to 3.
b. point 2 to 5.
c. point 1 to 4.
d. point 3 to 4.

118. A nurse is caring for a client who has just begun therapy with theophylline (Theo-24). The nurse will teach the client to limit the intake of which of the following while taking this medication?
a. cola, coffee, and chocolate
b. cream cheese, dairy creamer, and cottage cheese
c. lobster, shrimp, and crawfish
d. pineapple, oranges, and watermelon

119. The nurse is working with a client with a depersonalization disorder. The nurse plans care for a client with
a. fixed, lifelike, false beliefs.
b. loss of personal reality.
c. loss of recall of personal memories.
d. two or more distinctive personalities.

120. The nurse is caring for a client in the intensive care unit (ICU) with a basal skull fracture. Upon assessment, the nurse notes clear drainage from the client's right nares. Which of the following admission orders should the nurse question?
a. cold packs for facial bruising
b. head of bed elevated 30 degrees
c. insertion of a nasogastric tube
d. turning the client every two hours

121. The nurse assessing a young child observes the following. The nurse correctly documents this as

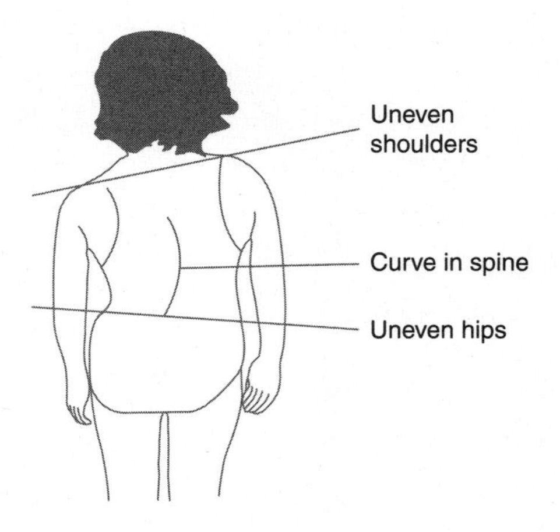

a. kyphosis
b. lordosis
c. scoliosis
d. Scheuermann's disease

122. The nurse is making rounds on a nursing unit and notices that smoke is coming from a client's room. Upon entering the client's room, the nurse notes the client is standing in the bathroom with his hospital gown on fire. Which of the following actions should the nurse take immediately?

a. Call a medical code.
b. Find the closest fire alarm box and activate it.
c. Obtain water from the client's bathroom and douse the client.
d. Tell the client to drop and roll on the floor.

123. Beractant was administered to a preterm infant. The nurse caring for the infant should monitor for which of the following adverse reactions?

a. bradycardia
b. necrotizing enterocolitis
c. retinopathy
d. tachycardia

124. A nurse is caring for a terminally ill client. The client's family is called to the hospital because the client's death is imminent. Which of the following assessment findings would lead the nurse to conclude that the client's death is near? Select all that apply.

1. Blood pressure is 80/60 mm Hg.
2. Body is rigid, and lack of change in position is noted.
3. Cheyne-Stokes respirations are documented.
4. The client's extremities are warm to the touch.
5. The client states he is dying.
6. The client reports seeing family members who have passed on.

a. 1, 2, 3, 4, 5, 6
b. 1, 2, 4, 6
c. 2, 3, 5, 6
d. 2, 4, 5

125. The nurse is admitting a client with an antisocial personality disorder. The highest-priority assessment for this client includes the client's risk for

a. delirium.
b. hallucinations.
c. harming self or others.
d. substance abuse.

126. A client is scheduled for a Schilling's test. The nurse will instruct the client to complete which of the following?

a. Administer a Fleets Enema the evening before the test.
b. Collect urine for 12 hours prior to the test.
c. Empty the bladder prior to the test.
d. Have nothing by mouth for eight hours prior to the test.

127. The nurse is developing a teaching plan for a seven-year-old child on the administration of insulin. The child seems unable to concentrate, fidgets, and interrupts the nurse during the teaching sessions. The nurse should

a. assess for history of ADHD.
b. check the child's blood sugar.
c. instruct the parents, not the child.
d. rely on written instructions.

128. The nurse is preparing to administer a blood transfusion. Which of the following nursing interventions is appropriate for the nurse to take when setting up the supplies for the transfusion?

a. Ensure the blood is left at room temperature for one hour prior to the infusion.
b. Add any required IV medication to the blood bag within a half hour of the planned infusion.
c. Prime the blood tubing set with 0.9% normal saline, completely filling the filter.
d. Use a small-bore catheter to prevent rapid infusion of blood products.

129. A nurse is planning care for a teenage pregnant girl. The nurse plans for the client's care knowing that teenage pregnancy places the client at risk for which of the following complications?
a. anemia
b. gestational diabetes
c. placenta previa
d. preterm delivery

130. The nurse is caring for a client who is suspected of experiencing an abdominal aortic aneurysm. Which of the following assessment findings will aid in confirming this diagnosis?
a. boardlike, rigid abdomen
b. knifelike pain in the back area
c. pulsating mass in the abdomen
d. unequal femoral pulses

131. A child with cerebral palsy has involuntary writhing motions. The nurse documents this as
a. athetosis.
b. ataxia.
c. hypertonia.
d. hypotonia.

132. A client is admitted to a medical-surgical unit with thrombophlebitis in the right leg. Five hours after admission to the unit, the client becomes confused and diaphoretic. Upon further assessment, the client is coughing up blood-streaked sputum and is complaining of severe chest pain on inspiration. Which of the following should the nurse do first?
a. Administer oxygen via nasal cannula.
b. Perform the Heimlich maneuver.
c. Position the client in a Fowler's position.
d. Place the client in the Trendelenburg position.

133. The nurse is assessing a client with dementia. To facilitate the assessment of cognition, the nurse should use which of the following?
a. CAGE
b. HITS
c. MMS
d. PSA

134. A telemetry nurse is analyzing the ECG rhythm strip of a client she is caring for. The nurse notes that there are nine QRS complexes in a six-second strip. The nurse calculates the client's heart rate as which of the following?
a. 54 bpm
b. 80 bpm
c. 88 bpm
d. 90 bpm

135. During a newborn assessment, the nurse observes that one half of the infant's skin is dark pink and the other is pale. The nurse documents this finding as
a. acrocyanosis.
b. harlequin changes.
c. lanugo.
d. milia.

136. The nurse is caring for a client with a head injury. The client has clear drainage from the nose and ears. How can the nurse determine if the drainage is cerebrospinal fluid (CSF)?
a. Measure the pH of the fluid.
b. Measure the specific gravity of the fluid.
c. Test the fluid for glucose.
d. Test the fluid for chloride.

137. The nurse is examining a teenager with anorexia nervosa. What might the nurse find during the history and assessment?
a. binge eating and purging
b. BMI less than 25
c. increased sodium levels
d. early onset of menses

138. An elderly female client presents to the community clinic stating foot pain. Upon further assessment, the client complains of "improperly fitting shoes and sore feet." The client additionally relays that her primary physician has referred her to a podiatrist. Based on the illustration, the nurse accurately identifies the client's bunion at which location?

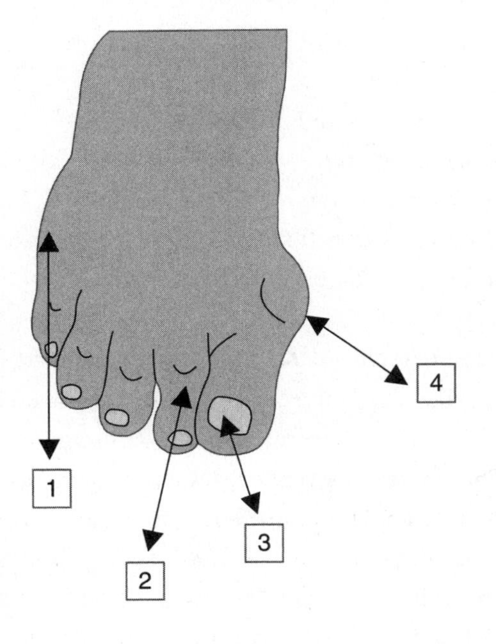

a. 1
b. 2
c. 3
d. 4

139. A client's labor is being augmented with oxytocin. The fetal monitor shows the fetal heart rate to be 170 with late decelerations. The nurse's first intervention should be:
a. Administer oxygen.
b. Contact the physician.
c. Place client in left lateral position.
d. Stop the oxytocin.

140. A client is admitted to the hospital with a detached retina of the right eye. The nurse patches both eyes. The client's family member asks, "Why are you patching both eyes?" The nurse's best response is:
a. "To decrease eye movement."
b. "To prevent eye infections."
c. "To prevent photophobia."
d. "To prevent nystagmus."

141. A client with a delusional disorder believes that her face has become disfigured even though it has not. The nurse knows that this belief is representative of which subtype of delusional disorder?
a. conjugal
b. erotomania
c. persecutory
d. somatic

142. The nurse is caring for a client diagnosed with liver failure. Which of the following laboratory values would the nurse expect to find?
a. decreased serum creatinine
b. decreased serum sodium
c. increased ammonia level
d. increased serum calcium

143. A father reports that his child's temperature is 102.5 Fahrenheit. This equates to how many degrees Celsius?

a. 29.17
b. 39.17
c. 40.94
d. 56.94

144. A 50-year-old male client is diagnosed with Laennec's cirrhosis. The client has extensive ascites and his respirations are rapid and shallow. The physician has decided to perform a paracentesis. The nurse caring for the client during this procedure will give highest priority to which of the following?

a. frequently obtaining the client's blood pressure (BP) and pulse during the procedure
b. gathering all the appropriate sterile equipment
c. positioning the client upright on the edge of the bed
d. properly labeling the abdominal fluid and sending it to the laboratory

145. The nurse is completing a newborn assessment when a swelling such as the following is noted:

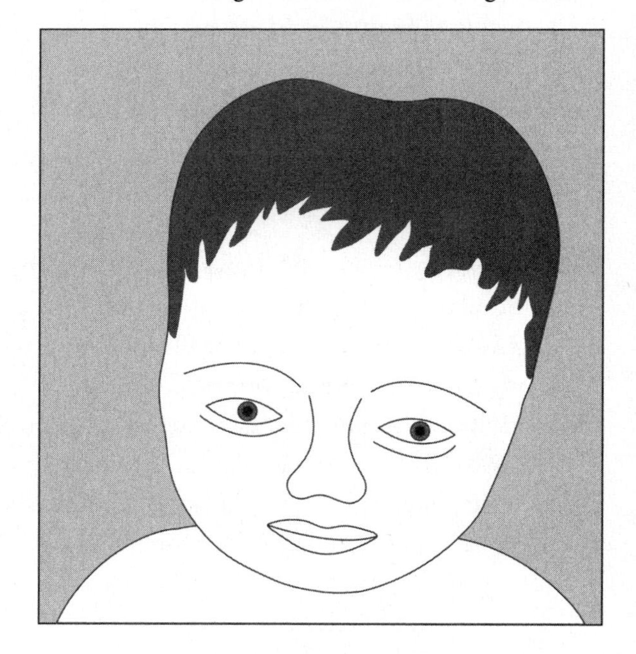

The nurse should document this as:

a. anencephaly
b. caput succedaneum
c. cephalohematoma
d. hydrocephalus

146. An emergency department nurse is caring for a male client injured in a motor vehicle collision (MVC). The nurse observes use of accessory muscles, severe chest pain, shortness of breath, and agitation. The nurse also notices one side of the client's chest moving differently from the other. The nurse suspects a flail chest. Based on these observations, which of the following is the nurse's best initial action?

a. Administer pain medication as prescribed.
b. Apply a sandbag to the flail side of the chest.
c. Prepare for intubation and mechanical ventilation.
d. Prepare for chest tube insertion.

147. The order for a teenage girl with asthma reads, "120 mg aminophylline (theophylline) p.o. b.i.d." The nurse has 80 mg per 15 ml solution of aminophylline available. How many teaspoons should the nurse administer?

a. 3
b. 3.5
c. 4
d. 4.5

148. A client is being treated in the emergency department (ED) after sustaining a fracture of the left tibia four hours ago. A long leg cast has been applied. Upon assessment, the client is complaining of increasing pain. The pain is more intense with passive flexion of the toes. The nurse suspects the client is developing compartment syndrome. Which of the following actions should the nurse take initially?

a. Administer the client's PRN narcotic medications for pain and reassess the client in 15 minutes.
b. Elevate the casted leg to the heart level, notify the physician, and prepare to split the cast.
c. Notify the physician and prepare the client for an emergency fasciotomy.
d. Raise the left leg above the heart, apply ice, and notify the physician.

149. A teenager was prescribed Percocet after arthroscopic knee surgery. The client takes the medication every four to six hours as prescribed. Two months later, the client is continuing to take the Percocet. The nurse documents the client's

a. dependency.
b. substance use.
c. tolerance.
d. withdrawal.

150. A client has just returned to the unit after having a femoral arteriogram completed. Which of the following assessments is essential for the nurse to complete initially?

a. auscultating the client's lung sounds
b. inspecting the client's groin area
c. palpating the client's carotid pulse
d. taking the client's blood pressure

151. The nurse is preparing to give a woman in preterm labor betamethasone (Celestone). The nurse plans to administer the medication as two intramuscular (IM) injections given

a. six hours apart.
b. 12 hours apart.
c. 24 hours apart.
d. 48 hours apart.

152. The nurse is caring for a client in the (ICU) following a craniotomy. The client has an intracranial pressure monitoring device in place. The client is becoming lethargic, and the nurse notes that the intracranial pressure reading is high. How should the nurse position the client?

a. Elevate the head of the bed (HOB) to a position that promotes optimal venous outflow for the client.
b. Elevate the head of the bed 90°. Position the client upright with pillows supporting the client's head.
c. Place the client flat in bed with his or her legs elevated 15 degrees on pillows.
d. Place the client in the left side lying position with pillows to support the client's back.

153. The nurse is examining a six-month-old infant. The nurse recommends to the physician that the infant may need further neurological screening based on the presence of which of the following findings?
a. palmar grasp
b. plantar grasp
c. sucking reflex
d. tonic neck reflex

154. A client had a cast applied to the left leg in the ED. The nurse has provided the client with discharge instructions. Which of the following statements indicates that the client understands the instructions?
a. "I will pack the left leg in ice for 24 hours to help the cast dry."
b. "I will place the casted leg on a fabric-covered pillow to help it dry."
c. "If my leg gets itchy, I can use a knitting needle to gently itch under the cast."
d. "When I get home, I will use my hair drier to help my cast dry faster."

155. The nurse is administering an ergot alkaloid to a client who had a postpartum hemorrhage. It is important for the nurse to monitor the client for
a. elevated blood pressure.
b. edema.
c. increased heart rate.
d. increased respirations.

156. The nurse is caring for a client who had a central line placed for IV fluid administration. When the nurse enters the client's room to reassess the client, the IV bag is empty, the IV line is full of air, and the client is dyspneic. Which of the following is the best initial action by the nurse?
a. Disconnect the IV tubing and place the client on the left side with the head down.
b. Call a code and begin CPR immediately.
c. Hang another IV bag as soon as possible, disconnect the IV tubing, and prime the line.
d. Notify the physician and administer oxygen via nasal cannula immediately.

157. A client is prescribed disulfiram (Antabuse). The nurse knows that this medication is used to treat
a. alcohol abuse.
b. anxiety.
c. delirium.
d. depression.

158. A nurse is caring for a client in the ICU who is receiving mechanical ventilation. The high-pressure alarm begins to sound repeatedly. The client is sleeping quietly. Which of the following is the most appropriate initial response by the nurse?
a. Call the respiratory therapist to assess the ventilator.
b. Check the ventilator tubing.
c. Obtain an arterial blood gas.
d. Reposition the client to stimulate coughing.

159. The nurse is assessing a child admitted to the emergency room for suspected appendicitis. Which of the following would the nurse expect to find? Select all that apply.
1. decreased white blood cells
2. periumbilical area pain
3. lower left quadrant abdominal pain
4. rebound tenderness

a. 1, 2
b. 1, 3
c. 2, 4
d. 3, 4

160. The nurse is caring for a client with a past medical history of seizures. While the nurse is performing morning care, the client begins to have a seizure. What is the priority assessment of the nurse at this time?
a. the length of the seizure activity
b. presence or absence of an aura
c. type and progression of seizure activity
d. events that precipitated the seizure activity

161. A client with anxiety states to the nurse that she knows something bad is going to happen. The client seems unable to focus on anything else. The nurse documents the client's anxiety as
a. mild.
b. moderate.
c. severe.
d. panic.

162. A 70-year-old male is admitted to the hospital with a diagnosis of gout. During the nurse's admission assessment to the unit, which of the following is the client most likely to report to the nurse?
a. a gradual onset of pain, swelling, redness, and warmth of the affected joint
b. a gradual onset of pain, swelling, redness, and warmth of the affected joint when walking
c. a recent history of trauma, alcohol ingestion, surgical stress, or illness
d. no recent alcohol consumption or dietary changes

163. The nurse administering magnesium sulfate determines that the client might be experiencing magnesium toxicity when which of the following is observed?
a. depressed patellar reflex
b. elevated blood pressure
c. increased respiratory rate
d. increased urinary output

164. An adult client is to receive Tazicef (ceftazidime) 500 mg IM (intramuscularly) q8 hours for diagnosis of pneumonia. A vial of the medication supplies 1 gram that needs to be reconstituted with 5 mL of diluent (sterile water). After the medication has been reconstituted, how much medication should the nurse withdraw into the syringe based on the illustration?

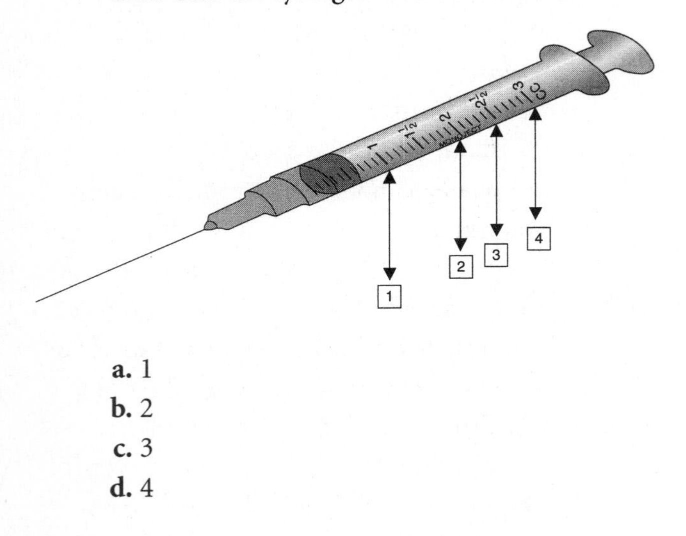

a. 1
b. 2
c. 3
d. 4

165. The nurse is planning to perform the Guthrie test on a child. The nurse knows that this test screens for

a. Down syndrome
b. Hip dysplasia
c. Lead toxicity
d. Phenylketonuria

Answers

1. a. The nurse should wear gloves upon entering the client's room. This is standard procedure when a client is ordered contact precautions. Choice **b** is incorrect. Gloves should also be worn in this instance; however, contact precautions require the nurse to wear gloves upon entering the room, not only when providing care within five feet of the client. Choice **c** is incorrect. Gloves should also be worn in this instance; however, contact precautions require the nurse to wear gloves upon entering the room, not only when anticipating a dressing change. Choice **d** is incorrect. Gloves should also be worn in this instance; however, contact precautions require the nurse to wear gloves upon entering the room, not only when the potential of contamination from body fluids exists.
Category: Safe and Effective Care Environment: Safety and Infection Control
Subcategory: Adult: Miscellaneous

2. b. A fetal heart rate of 120 per minute is within normal limits and therefore is not a sign of magnesium toxicity. Choice **a** is incorrect. Hypotonic and/or absent reflexes are signs of magnesium toxicity. Choice **c** is incorrect. One sign of magnesium toxicity is respiratory depression of < 12 per minute. Choice **d** is incorrect. Decreased urinary output such as < 30 cc/hour is a sign of magnesium toxicity.
Category: Physiological Integrity: Pharmacology and Parenteral Therapies
Subcategory: Maternal Infant: Maternal Medications

3. a. Atropine is a mydriatic and cycloplegic medication and is contraindicated in clients with glaucoma. This medication will dilate the pupil and can increase intraocular pressure in the eye. Choice **b** is incorrect. Betaxolol (Betoptic) is a miotic agent that is used to treat glaucoma. Choice **c** is incorrect. Pilocarpine (Ocusert Pilo-20) is a miotic agent that is used to treat glaucoma. Choice **d** is incorrect. Pilocarpine Hydrochloride (Isopto Carpine) is a miotic agent that is used to treat glaucoma.
Category: Physiological Integrity: Physiological Adaptation
Subcategory: Adult: Endocrine Disorders

4. d. The tonsils reach their maximum size between the ages of 10 and 12. Choices **a, b,** and **c** are incorrect. The tonsils do not reach their maximum size before the age of 10.
Category: Health Promotion and Maintenance
Subcategory: Pediatrics: Assessment

5. b. The Glasgow Coma Scale assesses eye opening (1), motor response (2), and verbal performance (4). Choice **a** is incorrect. Pupil reaction (3) is not part of the Glasgow Coma Scale. Choice **c** is incorrect. Motor response (2) is also part of the Glasgow Coma Scale. Choice **d** is incorrect. Pupil reaction (3) is not part of the Glasgow Coma Scale; eye opening (1) and verbal performance (4) are.
Category: Physiological Integrity: Physiological Adaptation
Subcategory: Adult: Neurological Disorders

6. b. Empathy is the ability to take another's perspective into consideration and communicate the understanding back to the person. Choice **a** is incorrect. Assertiveness involves stating your thoughts and feelings even when others may disagree. Choice **c** is incorrect. Sympathy involves harmony or agreement in the sharing of feelings of another. Choice **d** is incorrect. Transference involves the redirection of feelings from one person to another.
Category: Psychosocial Integrity
Subcategory: Mental Health: Therapeutic Communication

7. b. Consistency for mealtimes assists with regulation of blood glucose, so the best option is for the client to be returned to the unit to have lunch at the usual time. Choice **a** is incorrect. This is an intervention that is invasive, unnecessary, and not accompanied by a physician's order. Choice **c** is incorrect. This delay in eating may cause the client to experience hypoglycemia. Choice **d** is incorrect. A glass of milk or juice will keep the client from becoming hypoglycemic but will cause a sudden rise in blood glucose because of the rapid absorption of the simple carbohydrate in these items.
Category: Physiological Integrity: Pharmacology and Parenteral Therapies
Subcategory: Adult: Endocrine Disorders

8. c. Betamethasone is an antenatal glucocorticoid and is used to promote maturation of the fetal lungs. Choice **a** is incorrect. Betamethasone is used to promote fetal lung maturation. Examples of medications used to lower maternal blood pressure when the client is preeclampsic include labetalol and magnesium sulfate. Choice **b** is incorrect. Betamethasone is used to promote fetal lung maturation. Magnesium sulfate is used to prevent maternal seizures, but there are no medications to prevent fetal seizures. Choice **d** is incorrect. Betamethasone are used to promote fetal lung maturation. Tocolytic medications such as Brethine is used to stop premature maternal contractions.
Category: Physiological Integrity: Pharmacology and Parenteral Therapies
Subcategory: Maternal Infant: Maternal Medications

9. c. These foods are all permitted on a full liquid diet, but oatmeal is not. Choices **a**, **b**, and **d** is incorrect. All these foods are permitted on a full liquid diet.
Category: Physiological Integrity: Basic Care and Comfort
Subcategory: Adult: Gastrointestinal Disorders

10. b. Low birth rate and maternal smoking during pregnancy increase an infant's risk for SIDS. Choice **a** is incorrect. A low birth rate increases the infant's risk for SIDS, but sleeping with a pacifier reduces the risk for SIDS. Choice **c** is incorrect. Smoking during pregnancy does increase an infant's risk for SIDS. However, it is recommended that infants are placed on their back for sleep. Choice **d** is incorrect. It is recommended that infants be offered a pacifier for sleep as well as being placed on their back for sleep to decrease the incidence of SIDS.
Category: Physiological Integrity
Subcategory: Pediatrics: Respiratory Disorders

11. a. Hemianopsia is the loss of half of the visual field and is classified by the location of the missing visual field: the outer half (bitemporal), the same half (homonymous), the right half (right homonymous), the left half (left homonymous), the upper half (superior), or the lower half (inferior) of each visual field. This illustration demonstrates left homonymous hemianopsia, which is blindness in the temporal half of one eye and the nasal half of the other eye, occurring on the left side of each eye. Choice **b** is incorrect. This illustration demonstrates a normal visual field. Choice **c** is incorrect. Hemianopsia is the loss of half of the visual field and is classified by the location of the missing visual field. This illustration demonstrates right homonymous hemianopsia. Choice **d** is incorrect. This illustration demonstrates a visual field of a client diagnosed with glaucoma.
Category: Physiological Integrity: Reduction of Risk
Subcategory: Adult: Neurological Disorders

12. d. The first intervention by the nurse when a client experiences uterine atony in the postpartum period is to massage the fundus. Choice **a** is incorrect. To determine whether packed red blood cell administration is needed, the client's hemoglobin and hematocrit levels would first need to be assessed. Choice **b** is incorrect. The nurse should first massage the fundus. Then if the client is still experiencing uterine atony, pitocin might be ordered. Choice **c** is incorrect. If the client is experiencing uterine atony due to an overdistended bladder, insertion of a urinary catheter may assist in resolving the atony. However, the first intervention by the nurse for urine atony is always to massage the fundus. **Category:** Safe and Effective Care Management
Subcategory: Maternal Infant: Postpartum

13. d. When clients are receiving chemical sedation or restraints, they should be monitored closely for excessive drowsiness and/or respiratory depression. In situations when long-acting sedation is utilized, care must be taken as the effects of these medications are not seen for up to one hour after administration. Choice **a** is incorrect. The client may require physical restraints if the client is significantly agitated. However, in this scenario, there is no mention of additional restraints. Choice **b** is incorrect. The client may experience pain, and pain may also accompany restlessness. However, pain is not a side effect of chemical restraints. Choice **c** is incorrect. The client may experience an increase in blood pressure; however, hypertension should not occur from the administration of IV sedatives and thus is not considered a common side effect of chemical sedations and restraints.
Category: Safe and Effective Care Environment: Safety and Infection Control
Subcategory: Adult: Miscellaneous

14. c. This statement encourages the client to clarify and verbalize his or her feelings. Choice **a** is incorrect. The nurse should not leave the client alone, and this statement does not enable the client to verbalize feelings. Choice **b** is incorrect. This statement invalidates the client's feelings; additionally, insertion of an IV can be perceived as painful. Choice **d** is incorrect. This statement facilitates a power struggle between the client and the nurse. The client does have the right to refuse the insertion of an IV.
Category: Psychosocial Integrity
Subcategory: Mental Health: Therapeutic Communications

15. d. The client must be able to maintain a patent airway during the use of conscious sedation. Oversedation may result in loss of airway and resultant respiratory distress. Choice **a** is incorrect. The client may experience an allergic reaction due to sedation used; however, the loss of airway, resulting in respiratory distress, is a more common complication. Choice **b** is incorrect. A change or alteration in level of consciousness is not an expected side effect of conscious sedation. Choice **c** is incorrect. Hypertension is not a side effect associated with the use of conscious sedation.
Category: Physiological Integrity: Reduction of Risk
Subcategory: Adult: Cardiovascular Disorders

16. b. The bittersweet phase of grief occurs with reminders of the loss such as an anniversary date. During this time, the client typically experiences episodic bouts of sadness and crying. Choice **a** is incorrect. During the anticipatory stage of grief there is knowledge of the impending loss; the fetus is still alive but the prognosis is poor. Choice **c** is incorrect. During the intense phase of grief, there is deep sadness and symptoms of fatigue, headaches, dizziness, backaches, and insomnia. Guilt and anger may also be expressed. Choice **d** is incorrect. During the reorganization phase of grief, the client attempts to understand why the loss occurred. The client returns to daily activities at work and at home.
Category: Psychosocial Integrity
Subcategory: Maternal Infant: Maternal Complications

17. b. The client who is MRSA positive should be placed in a private room or a semiprivate room with a client with an active infection caused by the same organism. Choice **a** is incorrect. It is not necessary to place the client in a negative air pressure room; this intervention is included in airborne precautions and is not necessary for contact precautions. Choice **c** is incorrect. It is not necessary for nurses or other healthcare providers interacting with the client to wear an N-95 respirator. This intervention is associated with airborne precautions and is not necessary for contact precautions. Choice **d** is incorrect. It is not necessary for nursing staff or other healthcare providers interacting with the client to wear a mask. This intervention is associated with airborne precautions and is not necessary for contact precautions.
Category: Safe and Effective Care Environment: Safety and Infection Control
Subcategory: Adult: Miscellaneous

18. a. The nurse should expect the fontanels to be bulging due to an increased retention of cerebral spinal fluid in the ventricles of the brain. Choice **b** is incorrect. A firm fontanel is the expected finding in a healthy six-month-old. Hydrocephalus is an increased retention of cerebral spinal fluid within the ventricles of the brain. The increased pressure from the fluid would cause the fontanel to bulge. Choice **c** is incorrect. Hydrocephalus would cause increased intracranial pressure; therefore, the pulse would be expected to decrease while the blood pressure increased. Choice **d** is incorrect. A sunken fontanel would be expected in an infant who was dehydrated.
Category: Physiological Integrity: Physiological Adaptation
Subcategory: Pediatrics

19. c. This is a therapeutic and appropriate comment for the nurse to make. Sharing an observation with the client conveys awareness of the client's feelings and promotes further communication between the client and nurse. Choices **a**, and **b** are incorrect. They are not therapeutic and appropriate comments for the nurse to make. They don't recognize the feelings the client is undergoing. Choice **d** is incorrect. This is not a therapeutic and appropriate comment for the nurse to make. Asking why the client feels a certain way doesn't promote therapeutic communication.
Category: Psychosocial Integrity
Subcategory: Adult: Miscellaneous

20. a. By distracting the toddler with a book, the nurse gives the toddler attention and provides the toddler with an activity. The nurse will then be able to continue educating the eight-year-old without interruptions from the toddler. Choice **b** is incorrect. Toddlers are egocentric and demand attention. If ignored, the toddler will continue to seek attention through interruptions. Choice **c** is incorrect. The mother may not approve of the nurse reprimanding the child. Additionally, this may encourage the child to continue to interrupt for attention. Choice **d** is incorrect. This statement may offend the mother and does not offer any assistance to facilitate the toddler behaving in an appropriate manner.
Category: Psychosocial Integrity
Subcategory: Mental Health: Therapeutic Communications

21. c. Providing the specific information requested by the client comforts and reassures the client, who feels lost and confused, and promotes orientation. Choice **a** is incorrect. The nurse should not scold or infantilize the client. Choice **b** is incorrect. The nurse should not assume that the client will remember the name of the hospital after seeing the sign in the hallway. Choice **d** is incorrect. The nurse should not assume that a client with Alzheimer's disease will remember being admitted to the hospital, and should provide specific information about when the client's family will arrive.
Category: Psychosocial Integrity
Subcategory: Adult: Neurological Disorders

22. d. Methotrexate is administered as a single injection for unruptured ectopic pregnancies when the blastocyte is less than 3.5 cm in diameter. Choice **a** is incorrect. After a complete abortion, the nurse monitors for the client's serum HCG levels to return to prepregnancy levels, but would not administer methotrexate. Choice **b** is incorrect. Although methotrexate is a recommended treatment for ectopic pregnancies, it is contraindicated for ruptured tubal pregnancies. Choice **c** is incorrect. For threatened abortions, the client's treatment plan might include bed rest, avoidance of stress, and sedation, but not the administration of methotrexate.
Category: Safe and Effective Management of Care: Management of Care
Subcategory: Maternal Infant: Maternal Complications

23. a. The nurse should assess the second chamber of the chest tube drainage system. The second chamber is the water-seal chamber. Continuous bubbling in this chamber is unexpected and indicates a leak between the client and the water seal. The air leak could also be inside the client's thorax, at the chest tube insertion site, between tubing connections, or within the system. The nurse also needs to be aware that in a wet suction, constant gentle bubbling should occur in the first chamber (the suction-control chamber) when using suction. Choice **b** is incorrect. This area of the chest tube, the suction control, would not be assessed to determine if an air leak was present. Choice **c** is incorrect. This area of the chest tube, the actual tube itself, would not be assessed to determine if an air leak was present. Choice **d** is incorrect. This area of the chest tube, the fluid collection chamber, would not be assessed to determine if an air leak was present.
Category: Physiological Integrity: Reduction of Risk
Subcategory: Adult: Neurological Disorders

24. a. Solitary play is appropriate for an infant, that is, a child aged 1 to 12 months. Choice **b** is incorrect. Parallel play (playing alongside but not with another) is appropriate for a toddler. Choice **c** is incorrect. A preschooler engages in associative play (playing together but without group goals). Choice **d** is incorrect. School age children engage in cooperative play (play that follows organized rules with defined leaders and followers).
Category: Physiological Integrity: Basic Care and Comfort
Subcategory: Pediatrics: Developmental Milestones

25. d. The client should be instructed that the most appropriate time to apply the antiembolism stockings is before the client rises from bed in the morning. This will maximize the compression effect, thus lessening venous distention and development of edema. Choice **a** is incorrect. Even though the client is ambulating frequently, the antiembolism stockings should also be worn in an effort to prevent the development of thromboembolic disease. Choice **b** is incorrect. If the stockings begin to cause skin discomfort to the client, the stockings should be removed and the skin underneath must be assessed by the nursing staff. The nursing staff must ensure that the stockings are reapplied without twisting or wrinkles. Choice **c** is incorrect. The client should be instructed not to cross his or her legs. Crossing the legs impedes circulation and should be avoided with or without elastic stockings being in place.
Category: Physiological Integrity: Basic Care and Comfort
Subcategory: Adult: Cardiovascular Disorders

26. b. Using Naegele's rule, the nurse adds one year, subtracts three months, and adds seven days to the first day of the last menstrual period. Choice **a** is incorrect. To obtain a due date of January 9, 2013, the client's first day of the last menstrual period would have been April 2, 2012 (add one year; subtract three months and add seven days). Choice **c** is incorrect. To obtain a due date of January 23, 2013, the client's first day of the last menstrual period would have been April 16, 2012. Choice **d** is incorrect. To obtain a due date of January 26, 2013, the client's first day of the last menstrual period would have been April 19, 2012.
Category: Physiological Adaptation
Subcategory: Maternal Infant: Antepartum

27. b. Clients who are experiencing sleep deprivation often show signs of impaired cognitive functioning such as confusion. Choice **a** is incorrect. Cool extremities are not a sign or symptom associated with sleep deprivation. Choice **c** is incorrect. Depression is not a sign or symptom associated with sleep deprivation, but rather a cause. Choice **d** is incorrect. A period of apnea is not a sign or symptom associated with sleep deprivation.
Category: Physiological Integrity: Basic Care and Comfort
Subcategory: Adult: Cardiovascular Disorders

28. a. This is the best assertive response. The nurse stands up for herself. Choice **b** is incorrect. In this statement the nurse is negotiating or compromising what she wants with what the unit needs. It is not an assertive statement. Choice **c** is incorrect. Assertive statements do not begin with "you," as these statements put the emphasis on the other person's actions versus the nurse's feeling/wants/beliefs. Choice **d** is incorrect. This statement doesn't allow the nurse to stand up for herself, as assertive statements should. The nurse should stand up for herself by stating, "I cannot work the shift tonight."
Category: Safe and Effective Care Environment: Management of Care
Subcategory: Mental Health: Therapeutic Communications

29. a. The first action the nurse should complete is assess the client to ascertain if there are physical signs consistent with hypotension resulting in decreased perfusion of the brain and peripheral circulation. Choice **b** is incorrect. This nursing intervention is incorrect. The nurse should not elevate the head of the client's bed, as this action would further decrease the blood pressure. Choice **c** is incorrect. Only after assessing the client's present condition should the nurse recheck the blood pressure for accuracy of the reading. Choice **d** is incorrect. Determining the normal range of blood pressure is indicated after the assessment and verification of the reading is completed.
Category: Physiological Integrity: Reduction of Risk Potential
Subcategory: Adult: Cardiovascular Disorders

30. b. Only mild soaps or cleansing agents should be used to decrease irritation to the skin. Choice **a** is incorrect. The child's skin should be left moist to increase the effectiveness of ointments and/or creams to be applied after bathing. Choice **c** is incorrect. Warm, not hot, water should be used to promote and maintain hydration of the skin. Choice **d** is incorrect. The child should be lightly patted down with the towel to promote and maintain skin hydration and integrity.
Category: Health Promotion and Maintenance
Subcategory: Pediatrics: Assessment

31. a. The purpose of using a hypothermic blanket is to reduce the client's temperature, so the nurse should monitor the client for signs of hypothermia. Signs of hypothermia include bradycardia, hypotension, and drowsiness. The low cardiac output from hypotension (decrease in blood pressure) and bradycardia (slowing of the heart rate) affects the central nervous system, producing drowsiness. The client's urine output (5) is decreased in hypothermia as a result of decreased perfusion. Hypertension (3) (high blood pressure) and tachycardia (6) (an abnormally high heart rate) are not indicated in hypothermia. Choices **b**, **c**, and **d** are incorrect.
Category: Physiological Integrity: Physiological Adaptation
Subcategory: Adult: Miscellaneous

32. c. When the fetal head is one centimeter above the ischial spines, the client's station is documented as −1. Choice **a** is incorrect. Crowning occurs when the fetal head is at the opening of the fully effaced and dilated cervix. Choice **b** is incorrect. When the fetal head is level with the ischial spines, the client's station is documented as 0. Choice **d** is incorrect. When the fetal head is one centimeter below the ischial spines, the client's station is documented as +1.
Category: Safe and Effective Management of Care: Management of Care
Subcategory: Maternal Infant: Intrapartum

33. d. Compression of the oculomotor nerve will result in pupil dilation from the shifting of the brain and paralyzing the muscles controlling the pupillary size and shape. This is a neurological emergency, as herniation of the brain can occur; the physician should be notified immediately. Choice **a** is incorrect. A pupil size of 1, generally not included on the gauge, would not indicate increased intracranial pressure with compression of the oculomotor nerve. Choices **b** and **c** are incorrect. These pupil gauge sizes would not indicate increased intracranial pressure with compression of the oculomotor nerve.
Category: Physiological Integrity: Physiological Adaptation
Subcategory: Adult: Neurological Disorders

34. d. Developmental tasks are age-related. Choice **a** is incorrect. Development is a lifelong process; therefore development does not end in adolescence. Choices **b** and **c** are incorrect. Growth is cephalocaudal (head to feet) and proximodistal (center of the body outward).
Category: Physiological Integrity: Basic Care and Comfort
Subcategory: Pediatric Growth and Development

35. a. Clonidine is used to treat hypertension. The nurse should not apply a bioclusive, tegaderm, or tape to seal the patch, as it can affect the absorption of the medication. Choices **b**, **c**, and **d** are incorrect. These options follow correct procedure for applying a transdermal patch.
Category: Physiological Integrity: Pharmacology and Parenteral Therapies
Subcategory: Adult: Cardiovascular Disorders

36. d. Urinary output of at least 30 ml/hour is the most objective and least invasive assessment of adequate organ perfusion and oxygenation. Choice **a** is incorrect. A client experiencing hemorrhagic shock would have cool, clammy skin. Choice **b** is incorrect. Cyanosis in the buccal mucosa would be an indicator of inadequate organ and tissue oxygenation. Choice **c** is incorrect. Diminished restlessness is a subjective measure of organ perfusion and oxygenation.
Category: Safe and Effective Management of Care: Management of Care
Subcategory: Maternal Infant: Maternal Complications

37. b. The left dorsogluteal muscle is best located at position 2; above and outside a line drawn from the left posterior superior iliac spine to the left greater trochanter of the femur. The needle should be inserted at a 90-degree angle. Choices **a**, **c**, and **d** are incorrect. These locations are not correct.
Category: Physiological Integrity: Pharmacology and Parenteral Therapies
Subcategory: Adult: Miscellaneous

38. d. This statement allows the client to express his feelings, thoughts, and fears, an integral component of the therapeutic relationship. Choice **a** is incorrect. The nurse is not communicating honestly by stating the he or she does not know the results when the results are known. Trust is an integral component of the therapeutic relationship. Choice **b** is incorrect. This statement is untrue and disrupts trust within the therapeutic relationship. It also does not allow the client to discuss his feelings and fears. Choice **c** is incorrect. This is a false statement, as the nurse knows that the client has cancer. Trust is an integral component of the therapeutic relationship.
Category: Psychosocial Integrity
Subcategory: Mental Health: Therapeutic Communications

39. d. The nurse should be concerned with renal function, and urinary output provides information about renal functioning. Choices **a** and **b** are incorrect. The blood urea nitrogen (BUN) level and the creatinine clearance level also evaluate renal functioning, but they both require a physician order so may not be available for monitoring. Choice **c** is incorrect. Evaluating the client's fluid intake will not help determine whether the client is experiencing nephrotoxicity.
Category: Physiological Integrity: Pharmacology and Parenteral Therapies
Subcategory: Adult: Renal Disorders

40. a. A respiratory rate of 24 breaths per minute is within the normal range for a six-year-old boy; therefore, the nurse should document the apical rate. Choice **b** is incorrect. A respiratory rate of 24 breaths per minute in a six-year-old boy is considered within the normal limits; therefore, there is no need for another nurse to recheck the respirations. Choice **c** is incorrect. As the respiratory rate is within the normal limits for a six-year-old boy, the physician does not need to be notified. Choice **d** is incorrect. As the respiratory rate is within the normal limits for a six-year-old boy, the nurse does not need to recheck it.
Category: Health Promotion and Maintenance
Subcategory: Pediatrics: Assessment

41. **d.** The asterixis, a condition indicating this type of hand movement, indicates that the client has hepatic encephalopathy, and hepatic coma may occur. Choice **a** is incorrect. The ascites and weight gain do indicate the need for treatment but not as urgently as the changes in neurologic status. Choice **b** is incorrect. The upper right quadrant abdominal pain is not unusual for the client with cirrhosis, and does not require a change in treatment. Choice **c** is incorrect. Spider angiomas, such as described in this response, are not unusual for the client with cirrhosis, and do not require a change in treatment.
Category: Physiological Integrity: Physiological Adaptation
Subcategory: Adult: Gastrointestinal Disorders

42. **c.** Leopold's maneuver is used to assess the fetal presentation on a pregnant client. Choice **a** is incorrect. Chadwick's sign is a bluish discoloration of the uterus during pregnancy. Choice **b** is incorrect. Hegar's sign is a softening of the pregnant client's cervix that is noted during bimanual exam. Choice **d** is incorrect. McMurray's test is used to assess for a meniscal tear.
Category: Physiological Integrity: Basic Care and Comfort
Subcategory: Maternal Infant: Antepartum

43. **b.** The client is asking for more time to see his son's graduation, an example of a typical strategy in the bargaining phase. Choice **a** is incorrect. In the anger phase, the client may express anger at God or at healthcare professionals that he has cancer. Choice **c** is incorrect. In the denial phase, the client rejects the terminal diagnosis. Choice **d** is incorrect. While the client may exhibit symptoms of depression due to the terminal diagnosis, depression is not a phase of Kübler-Ross's stages of death and dying.
Category: Physiological Integrity: Basic Care and Comfort
Subcategory: Mental Health

44. **c.** Spironolactone is a potassium-sparing diuretic. Clients should be instructed to choose low-potassium foods such as apple juice rather than foods that have higher levels of potassium, such as citrus fruits. Choice **a** is incorrect. The fat content of the cheese is not relevant; thus the client does not have to consume only low-fat cheese. Choice **b** is incorrect. Clients should be taught to avoid salt substitutes, which are high in potassium. Choice **d** is incorrect. Because the client is using spironolactone as a diuretic, the nurse will encourage the client to increase fluid intake. Six glasses of water are not sufficient; the client should drink eight or more glasses of water each day.
Category: Physiological Integrity: Pharmacology and Parenteral Therapy
Subcategory: Adult: Cardiovascular Disorders

45. c. Symptoms of preeclampsia include +1 protein in the urine and blood pressure of 140/90 to 160/110. Choice **a** is incorrect. Eclampsia is characterized by the onset of seizure activity in a woman diagnosed with preeclampsia who did not have a history of seizures prior to pregnancy. Choice **b** is incorrect. Gestational hypertension is characterized by onset of hypertension without proteinuria that occurs after 20 weeks of pregnancy. Choice **d** is incorrect. Severe preeclampsia is characterized by the presence of any of the following in a woman diagnosed with preeclampsia: systolic blood pressure > 160, diastolic blood pressure > 110, +2 or +3 proteinuria, oliguria, epigastric pain, and elevated liver enzymes.
Category: Safe and Effective Care Management: Management of Care
Subcategory: Maternal Infant: Maternal Complications

46. a. The BMI calculation is:

$$\text{BMI} = (\text{Weight} \div \text{Height}^2) \times 703$$
$$= (160 \div 66^2) \times 703$$
$$= 25.8$$

Choices **b**, **c**, and **d** are incorrect.
Category: Safe and Effective Care Environment: Health Promotion and Maintenance
Subcategory: Adult: Miscellaneous

47. c. At seven to nine months of age, infants are able to smile at their mirror image. Choice **a** incorrect. At zero to three months infants are able to smile socially at another person. Choice **b** is incorrect. At four to six months of age, infants are able to discriminate strangers from parents. Choice **d** is incorrect. At 10 to 12 months of age, infants are increasingly aware of strangers.
Category: Health Promotion and Maintenance
Subcategory: Pediatrics: Growth and Development

48. a. A stage 3 ulcer involves full-thickness damage. This includes skin loss of the dermis and epidermis and penetration as far down as the subcutaneous tissue. Choices **b** and **c** are incorrect. This area, the dermis, does not indicate a stage 3 pressure ulcer. Choice **d** is incorrect. This area, the epidermis, does not indicate a stage 3 pressure ulcer.
Category: Safe and Effective Care Environment: Management of Care
Subcategory: Adult: Integumentary Disorders

49. a. The "B" in the SBAR communication technique stands for "background information." In this example the background is that the client is 79 years old and has a history of anxiety. Choice **b** is incorrect. This statement represents the "S," which stands for "situation" in the SBAR technique. Choice **c** is incorrect. This statement represents the "R," which stands for "recommendations" in the SBAR technique. Choice **d** is incorrect. This statement represents the "A" for "assessment" in the SBAR technique.
Category: Safe and Effective Care Environment: Safety and Infection Control
Subcategory: Mental Health: Anxiety Disorders

50. c. Ginkgo is useful in the prevention and treatment of dementia and cerebral insufficiency; thus, monitoring attention span would be appropriate. Choice **a** is incorrect. Assessing the client's blood pressure would not be helpful in determining the effectiveness of the ginkgo. Choice **b** is incorrect. Assessing the client's level of motivation would not be helpful in determining the effectiveness of the ginkgo. Choice **d** is incorrect. Evaluating the client's red blood cell count would not be helpful in determining the effectiveness of the ginkgo.
Category: Physiological Integrity: Pharmacology and Parenteral Therapy
Subcategory: Adult: Neurological Disorders

51. b. Hegar's sign is the softening of the cervix in pregnant women. Choice **a** is incorrect. Chadwick's sign is a bluish discoloration of the uterus in pregnant women. Choice **c** is incorrect. Homan's sign is pain elicited in the calf when the healthcare professional flexes the client's foot. Choice **d** is incorrect. Murphy's sign tests for gallbladder disease. It is elicited by asking the client to breathe deeply while palpating the costal margin of the upper right abdominal quadrant. If the gallbladder is inflamed, the client will experience pain.
Category: Health Promotion and Maintenance
Subcategory: Maternal Infant: Antepartum

52. a. The nurse will administer pain medication based on the principles of beneficence and nonmaleficence. Under these principles, the goal of pain management in a terminally ill client is adequate pain relief even if the effect of pain medications could hasten death. Choice **b** is incorrect. The client requires around-the-clock administration of pain medication to ensure that the client does not experience breakthrough pain and discomfort. Choice **c** is incorrect. Administration of analgesics on a PRN basis will not provide the consistent level of analgesia the client requires. Choice **d** is incorrect. The nurse should not rely on the client's family to request pain medication. Clients usually do not require so much pain medication that they are oversedated and unaware of stimuli.
Category: Safe and Effective Care Environment: Management of Care
Subcategory: Adult: Oncology Disorders

53. b. In stage 2 pressure ulcers, there is partial-thickness loss of the dermis presenting as a shallow wound with a red or pink wound bed. Choice **a** is incorrect. A stage 1 pressure ulcer is an area of intact erythema that does not blanch with pressure. Choice **c** is incorrect. A stage 3 pressure ulcer has full-thickness loss of the dermis. Subcutaneous tissue may be visible but not bone, tendon, or muscle. Choice **d** is incorrect. In stage 4 pressure ulcers, there is muscle, tendon, or bone visible.
Category: Physiological Integrity
Subcategory: Pediatrics

54. d. The nurse should implement the RICE treatment (rest, ice, compression, elevation) for soft tissue injuries. Use of a compression bandage around the ankle will decrease tissue swelling. Choice **a** is incorrect. The nurse should apply a cold compress, not a warm compress. Cold packs should be applied for the first 24 hours to reduce swelling. Choice **b** is incorrect. Moving the ankle through range of motion (ROM) activities will increase swelling and risk further injury. Choice **c** is incorrect. The football cleat does not need to be removed immediately and will help to compress the injury if it is left in place.
Category: Physiological Integrity: Reduction of Risk
Subcategory: Adult: Musculoskeletal Disorders

55. a. A closed posterior fontanel on a newborn infant is a sign of potential distress. Choice **b** is incorrect. The normal heart rate for a newborn is 120 to 160. Choice **c** is incorrect. The anterior fontanel of a newborn should be palpable. Choice **d** is incorrect. The normal respiratory rate for a newborn is 30 to 50.
Category: Physiological Integrity: Risk Reduction
Subcategory: Maternal Infant: Neonate Assessment

56. b. The client should first be placed in a semi-Fowler's position to maintain a patent airway and reduce incisional swelling. The blood-tinged secretions may obstruct the airway, so suctioning the client is the next appropriate action. Then the Hemovac should be drained because the 250 mL of drainage will decrease the amount of suction in the Hemovac and could lead to incisional swelling and poor healing. Last, the nasogastric (NG) tube should be reconnected to suction to prevent gastric dilation, nausea, and vomiting. Choices **a**, **c**, and **d** are incorrect. These sequences of events are not correct. See answer choice **b** for the correct sequence.
Category: Physiological Integrity: Physiological Adaptation
Subcategory: Adult: Respiratory Disorders

57. c. During the termination phase, the client may exhibit signs of anxiety or regression but is able to demonstrate satisfaction and competence. Choices **a** and **b** are incorrect. During the initiating/orienting phase the nurse begins to build trust and rapport. Choice **d** is incorrect. During the working phase, the focus is on mutually reaching set goals; coping mechanisms are identified and alternative behaviors are explored.
Category: Physiological Integrity: Basic Care and Comfort
Subcategory: Mental Health: Therapeutic Communications

58. d. The nurse should report the low white blood cell (WBC) count to the healthcare provider. Neutropenia places the client at risk for severe infection and is an indication that the chemotherapy dose may need to be lower or that WBC growth factors such as filgrastim (Neupogen) are needed. Neupogen is a prescription medication used to reduce the risk of infection in clients with some tumors who are receiving strong chemotherapy, which decreases the number of infection-fighting white blood cells. Choices **a**, **b**, and **c** are incorrect. These laboratory data do not indicate an immediate life-threatening adverse effect of the chemotherapy.
Category: Physiological Integrity: Reduction of Risk
Subcategory: Adult: Oncology Disorders

59. d. A sunken or depressed fontanel is a sign of dehydration. Choice **a** is incorrect. If the child's fontanel was bulging, it would indicate increased intercranial pressure. Choice **b** is incorrect. A closed fontanel in a 13-month-old child would be a part of normal growth and development, as the fontanel closes between 7 and 19 months of age, and therefore would not assist the nurse is determining whether the child was dehydrated. Choice **c** is incorrect. A firm anterior fontanel would be considered within the normal limits; a depressed or sunken fontanel would indicate dehydration.
Category: Physiological Integrity: Reduction of Risk
Subcategory: Pediatrics

60. d. The client will be required to stay in the hospital for several weeks following the procedure. The client requires strict protective isolation to prevent infection for two to four weeks after HSCT while waiting for the transplanted marrow to start generating cells. Choice **a** is incorrect. The HSCT takes place one or two days after chemotherapy to prevent damage to the transplanted cells by the chemotherapy drugs. Choice **b** is incorrect. This is inaccurate information. The transplanted cells are infused through an IV line; thus the transplant is not painful. Choice **c** is incorrect. This is inaccurate information. The procedure does not need to occur in an operating room.
Category: Physiological Integrity: Physiological Adaptation
Subcategory: Adult: Oncology Disorders

61. b. A score of 1 would indicate the neonate's central skin color was pink while the extremities were blue. Choice **a** is incorrect. A score of 0 would indicate the neonate's color was pale. Choice **c** is incorrect. A score of 2 would indicate that the neonate's skin color was pink both centrally and in the extremities. Choice **d** is incorrect. Scores for skin color on the Apgar scale range from 0 to 2, with 0 indicating a pale color, 1 indicating pink central color and blue extremities, and 2 indicating the skin color as pink throughout.
Category: Physiological Integrity: Physiological Adaptation
Subcategory: Maternal Infant: Neonate Assessment

62. d. The nurse should be certain that the client restricts free water intake. SIADH causes water retention, which leads to hyponatremia, so water intake is restricted. Choice **a** is incorrect. Ambulating the client may be included in the plan of care for any hospitalized client, but is not specifically indicated for the diagnosis of SIADH. Choice **b** is incorrect. Instructing the client to utilize incentive spirometry may be included in the plan of care for any hospitalized client, but is not specifically indicated for the diagnosis of SIADH. Choice **c** is incorrect. The nurse should monitor intake and output, but hourly monitoring is not required.
Category: Physiological Integrity: Physiological Adaptation
Subcategory: Adult: Endocrine Disorders

63. b. Clients with borderline personality disorder generally do not exhibit persistent feelings of mistrust toward others; rather, they tend to fluctuate in their emotions about other people. Choice **a** is incorrect. Clients with borderline personality disorder do exhibit impulsive behavior. Choice **c** is incorrect. Clients with borderline personality disorder often exhibit low self-esteem. Choice **d** is incorrect. Clients with borderline personality disorder often also have an issue with substance abuse.
Category: Psychosocial Integrity
Subcategory: Mental Health: Personality Disorders

64. d. Correct administration of KCL IV includes: Peripheral line: Usual concentration: 20 to 40 mEq/L; maximum: 80 mEq/L, infused at a maximum rate of 10 mEq/hour. Central line: Usual concentration: 20 to 60 mEq/L, infused at a maximum rate of 20 mEq/hour. Choice **a** is incorrect. The rate of administration, not the amount of KCL added to IV fluids, must be considered by the nurse. Choice **b** is incorrect. Rapid IV administration of KCL can cause cardiac arrest; KCL is administered at a maximal rate of 20 mEq/hr. Choice **c** is incorrect. KCL can cause inflammation of peripheral veins when administered peripherally, but it can be administered by this route.
Category: Physiological Integrity: Pharmacology and Parenteral Therapies
Subcategory: Adult: Fluid and Electrolyte Imbalances

65. c. Fine motor expectations for an eight-month-old include utilization of the pincer grasp, which involves the thumb and forefinger. Choice **a** is incorrect. Fine motor expectations for a one-month-old include opening and closing hands. Choice **b** is incorrect. Fine motor expectations for a four-month-old include transferring objects from one hand to the other. Choice **d** is incorrect. Fine motor expectations for an 11-month-old include scribbling.
Category: Health Promotion and Maintenance
Subcategory: Pediatrics: Developmental Milestones

66. **b.** Postoperative cataract surgery clients usually experience little or no pain, so a pain score of 6 out of 10 may indicate complications such as hemorrhage, infection, or increased intraocular pressure. Choices **a, c,** and **d** are incorrect. The information given by the client indicates a need for client teaching, but does not indicate that complications of the surgery may be occurring.
Category: Physiological Integrity: Physiological Adaptation
Subcategory: Adult: Eye and Ear Disorders

67. **a.** The head circumference of a one-week-old infant is expected to be 2 to 3 cm larger than the chest circumference. Choice **b** is incorrect. If the head circumference is larger than the chest circumference by 4 to 5 cm, this could be an indication of hydrocephalus. Choices **c** and **d** are incorrect. If the head circumference is smaller than the chest circumference by 2 cm or more, this could be an indication of an underdeveloped brain.
Category: Physiological Integrity: Health Promotion and Maintenance
Subcategory: Maternal Infant: Neonate Assessment

68. **d.** A darkened, quiet room will decrease the symptoms of the acute attack of Ménière's disease. Choice **a** is incorrect. Fluids are administered intravenously during an acute attack; thus the need to encourage an increase in oral fluids is not necessary. Choices **b** and **c** are incorrect. The client should be positioned for comfort.
Category: Physiological Integrity: Physiological Adaptation
Subcategory: Adult: Eye and Ear Disorders

69. **b.** The HPV vaccine is approved for females ages 9 to 25, but the CDC recommends that girls receive the vaccine between the ages of 10 and 12. Choice **a** is incorrect. The HPV vaccine is approved for use in females between the ages of 9 and 25. Choice **c** is incorrect. While the HPV vaccine is approved for females between the ages of 9 and 25, it is recommended that they receive it between the ages of 10 and 12. Choice **d** is incorrect. While the HPV vaccine is approved for females between the ages of 9 and 25, it is recommended that they receive the vaccine before becoming sexually active.
Category: Physiological Integrity: Reduction of Risk
Subcategory: Pediatrics: Assessment

70. **c.** Cervical spine injuries are commonly associated with electrical burns; therefore, stabilization of the cervical spine takes precedence after airway management. Choices **a**, **b**, and **d** are incorrect. These actions are included in the emergent care after electrical burns, but the most important priority is to avoid spinal cord injury.
Category: Physiological Integrity: Physiological Adaptation
Subcategory: Adult: Integumentary Disorders

71. **b.** Alcohol withdrawal symptoms include an elevated, not decreased, heart rate. Choice **a** is incorrect. Agitation is an early symptom of alcohol withdrawal. Choice **c** is incorrect. Hyperalertness is an early symptom of alcohol withdrawal. Choice **d** is incorrect. Seizures can occur during alcohol withdrawal, especially in the first 7 to 48 hours.
Category: Physiological Integrity: Reduction of Risk
Subcategory: Mental Health: Alcohol Withdrawal

72. c. CPAP therapy is very effective in improving sleep quality in clients with sleep apnea; however, many clients are noncompliant with the therapy. The nurse should be sure that the client is actually using the CPAP machine as prescribed. Choice **a** is incorrect. When CPAP is used as prescribed, the effects on sleep quality are seen immediately. Choice **b** is incorrect. Surgery may be an appropriate therapy for the client; however, suggesting surgery would not be an appropriate first action by the nurse in this situation. Choice **d** is incorrect. Utilizing a higher pressure setting will make it more difficult for the client to exhale and is likely to decrease client compliance with therapy.
Category: Physiological Integrity: Physiological Adaptation
Subcategory: Adult: Respiratory Disorders

73. c. This is a picture of a low-lying placenta previa. Choice **a** is incorrect. This is a picture of a marginal placenta previa. Choice **b** is incorrect. This is a picture of a complete placenta previa. Choice **d** is incorrect. This is a picture of a normally implanted placenta.
Category: Safe and Effective Management of Care: Management of Care
Subcategory: Maternal Infant: Maternal Complications

74. b. The abbreviations "qd" (daily)(order 1), "u"(units)(order 4), and "MS" (morphine sulfate)(order 5) are inappropriate abbreviations for a physician to use when writing a medication order. These abbreviations are prohibited by the Joint Commission. Orders 2 and 3 contain essential components of the medication order (i.e., medication name, dose, frequency, and route) and use acceptable abbreviations. Choices **a**, **c**, and **d** are incorrect. See answer choice **b.**
Category: Physiological Integrity: Pharmacology and Parenteral Therapies
Subcategory: Adult: Miscellaneous

75. a. Drooling can result from the ingestion of a corrosive substance. Choice **b** is incorrect. Jaundice is associated with acetaminophen overdose/poisoning. Choice **c** is incorrect. Oliguria is associated with acetylsalicylic overdose/poisoning. Choice **d** is incorrect. Tinnitus is associated with acetylsalicylic toxicity/poisoning.
Category: Physiological Integrity: Pharmacologic and Parenteral Therapies
Subcategory: Pediatrics: Gastrointestinal Disorders

76. b. Aromatherapy is used for stress reduction, and a decrease in the client's blood pressure and pulse would indicate that the aromatherapy was effective. Choice **a** is incorrect. Auscultating the client's breath sounds would not be used to determine the effectiveness of aromatherapy. Choice **c** is incorrect. Checking the incision for signs of infection would not be used to determine the effectiveness of aromatherapy. Choice **d** is incorrect. Monitoring the client's intake and output would not be used to determine the effectiveness of aromatherapy.
Category: Psychosocial Integrity
Subcategory: Adult: Miscellaneous

77. a. The monitor strip shows that the fetal heart rate is within the normal range in response to maternal contractions. The nurse should continue to monitor the client. Choice **b** is incorrect. There is no need to notify the physician at this point in time as the monitor strip does not indicate fetal distress. Choice **c** is incorrect. While the left lateral position promotes fetal blood flow and oxygenation, the monitor strip does not indicate fetal distress; therefore, the client does not need to be placed in the left lateral position. Choice **d** is incorrect. There is no indication of fetal distress on the monitor strip; therefore, the client will not need a cesarean section at this time.
Category: Physiological Integrity: Basic Care and Comfort
Subcategory: Maternal: Fetal Assessment

78. a. The client is demonstrating proper technique when elbows are bent at a 30° angle, indicating the use of the walker at the proper height for the client. Choice **b** is incorrect. This demonstrates improper technique: the client should stand erect while using the walker. Choice **c** is incorrect. This demonstrates improper technique: the client cannot be ambulating with partial weight bearing if the client lifts the walker off the floor. Choice **d** is incorrect. This demonstrates improper technique: the client cannot be ambulating with partial weight bearing while using a walker with four wheels.
Category: Physiological Integrity: Basic Care and Comfort
Subcategory: Adult: Musculoskeletal Disorders

79. a. Symptoms of cocaine overdose include cardiac arrhythmias, which can lead to cardiac arrest. Choice **b** is incorrect. Panic is associated with overdoses of hallucinogens such as LSD and PCP but not cocaine. Choice **c** is incorrect. Psychosis is associated with overdoses of hallucinogens such as LSD and PCP but not cocaine. Choice **d** is incorrect. Overdoses of opioids such as morphine and heroin place the client at risk for respiratory arrest.
Category: Physiological Integrity: Reduction of Risk
Subcategory: Mental Health: Substance Abuse

80. c. The purpose of using lactulose in a client with cirrhosis is to lower ammonia levels and prevent encephalopathy. Symptoms of a high ammonia level include confusion or extreme sleepiness. Hepatic encephalopathy is the occurrence of confusion, altered level of consciousness, and coma as a result of liver failure. In the advanced stages it is called hepatic coma. Choice **a** is incorrect. Although administration of lactulose may prevent constipation, the medication is not ordered for this purpose for this client. Choice **b** is incorrect. The medication is not ordered for this purpose for this client. Choice **d** is incorrect. Although administration of lactulose may prevent fluid loss via stool, the medication is not ordered for this purpose for this client.
Category: Physiological Integrity: Pharmacology and Parenteral Therapies
Subcategory: Adult: Gastrointestinal Disorders

81. d. Due to the risk for dehydration from vomiting, the nurse should include assessment for dehydration and documentation of intake and output in the client's plan of care. Choice **a** is incorrect. The child with pyloric stenosis is at risk for dehydration from vomiting, so an assessment of dehydration should be included in the plan of care. However, administration of blood products is not indicated. Choice **b** is incorrect. While an assessment for dehydration due to vomiting should be made, chelation therapy, which is utilized for lead poisoning, should not be administered. Choice **c** is incorrect. Administration of blood products is not indicated, and chelation therapy is used to treat lead poisoning.
Category: Physiological Integrity: Physiological Adaptation
Subcategory: Pediatrics: Gastrointestinal Disorders

82. a. This image represents a lobectomy, in which only a lobe of the lung is removed. Choice **b** is incorrect. This image demonstrates a pneumonectomy, in which the entire lung is removed. Choice **c** is incorrect. This image demonstrates a wedge resection, in which a small, well-circumscribed lesion is removed without regard for the location of the intersegmental planes. Choice **d** is incorrect. This image demonstrates a segmentectomy. Bronchopulmonary segments are subdivisions of the lung that function as individual units.
Category: Physiological Integrity: Physiological Adaptation
Subcategory: Adult: Oncology Disorders

83. d. Pregnant women should avoid soft cheeses such as feta and brie due to the potential for contracting listeria. Choice **a** is incorrect. Only undercooked eggs such as those with a running yolk need to be avoided during pregnancy. Choice **b** is incorrect. As long as the client does not consume more than 300 mg of caffeine per day, a cup of coffee in the morning is allowed. Choice **c** is incorrect. As long as the shrimp is cooked, it is safe to eat during pregnancy. Swordfish, shark, tilefish, and king mackerel should be avoided due to high levels of mercury they contain.
Category: Physiological Integrity: Risk Reduction
Subcategory: Maternal Infant: Antepartum

84. d. If the nurse experiences resistance during the insertion of the nasogastric tube, the nurse should remove the tube and try the other nares to prevent damage to nasal mucosa and internal structures. Choice **a** is incorrect. Asking the client to swallow water may help advance the tube, but will not prevent injury to the client. Choice **b** is incorrect. The tube has met resistance as it was being inserted; therefore checking for placement is inappropriate since it hasn't reached the stomach yet. Choice **c** is incorrect. The nurse should not continue to advance or push the tube into the nares, as this may injure the client.
Category: Physiological Integrity: Basic Care and Comfort
Subcategory: Adult: Gastrointestinal Disorders

85. **a.** Anticholinergic medications, which affect the central and peripheral nervous systems, are contraindicated with donepezil (Aricept). Choice **b** is incorrect. Diuretics may be contraindicated with certain types of kidney diseases, but not with acetylcholinesterase inhibitors, an example of which is Aricept. Choice **c** is incorrect. Narcotics should be use with caution for clients with respiratory conditions, but are not contraindicated for use with acetylcholinesterase inhibitors, an example of which is Aricept. Choice **d** is incorrect. Antipsychotic medications may cause neuroleptic malignant syndrome as an adverse reaction but are not contraindicated with alcetylcholinesterase inhibitors, an example of which is Aricept.
Category: Physiological Integrity: Pharmacology and Parenteral Therapies
Subcategory: Mental Health: Medications

86. **d.** A partial thromboplastin time (PTT) of 60 seconds is therapeutic for a client receiving heparin. The 60 seconds value falls within the therapeutic range of 1.5 to 2.5 times the control when a client is on heparin. The normal range of a PTT is 25 to 38 seconds. Choice **a** is incorrect. A phosphorus level is not used to measure the therapeutic effects of heparin therapy. The normal phosphorus level is 2.5 to 4.5 mg/dL. Choice **b** is incorrect. A platelet count is not used to measure the therapeutic effects of heparin therapy. The normal platelet level is 150,000 to 450,000/mm^3. Choice **c** is incorrect. A prothrombin time (PT) level is not used to measure the therapeutic effects of heparin therapy. The normal PT level is 11 to 13.5 seconds. A PT level is utilized to evaluate the effects of warfarin (Coumadin).
Category: Physiological Integrity: Reduction of Risk
Subcategory: Adult: Neurological Disorders

87. **d.** During the taking-hold phase, the mother feels in control; she is ready to begin caring for the infant and is receptive to learning infant care. Choice **a** is incorrect. During the letting-go phase the mother may feel role conflict about being a mother. Therefore, she may not be receptive to learning infant care. Choice **b** is incorrect. There is not a "letting-in" phase in Rubin's phases of bonding. Choice **c** is incorrect. During the taking-in phase, the mother is focused on her own needs and on her delivery experience and may not be receptive to learning infant care.
Category: Psychosocial Integrity
Subcategory: Maternal Infant: Postpartum

88. **a.** Guillain-Barré syndrome can cause respiratory acidosis, because the syndrome can affect the muscles of respiration, which might decrease alveolar ventilation and result in the retention of carbon dioxide. Choice **b** is incorrect. This client is at risk for developing metabolic acidosis. Choice **c** is incorrect. This client is at risk for developing metabolic alkalosis. Choice **d** is incorrect. This client is at risk for developing respiratory alkalosis.
Category: Physiological Integrity: Physiological Adaptation
Subcategory: Adult: Fluid and Electrolyte Imbalances

89. b. A decreased pulse coupled with increased blood pressure can be indications of increased intercranial pressure. Choice **a** is incorrect. A decreased pulse can indicate increased intercranial pressure, but the blood pressure would be increased, not decreased. Choice **c** is incorrect. Signs of increased intercranial pressure include increased blood pressure but the pulse would be decreased, not increased. Choice **d** is incorrect. Neither increased pulse nor decreased blood pressure is a symptom of increased intercranial pressure.
Category: Safe and Effective Care Environment: Management of Care
Subcategory: Pediatrics: Neurologic Conditions

90. c. Removing a client's spleen predisposes the client to an increased risk of developing an infection. Choice **a** is incorrect. There is not an increased risk of developing anemia following a splenectomy. Choice **b** is incorrect. There is not an increased risk of developing bleeding tendencies following a splenectomy. Choice **d** is incorrect. There is not an increased risk of developing lymphedema following a splenectomy.
Category: Physiological Integrity: Reduction of Risk
Subcategory: Adult: Hematological Disorders

91. a. There is no clinical significance to a client trembling during or after the third stage of delivery. Choices **b** and **c** are incorrect. While trembling can indicate fear in some situations, it does not have clinical significance when it occurs during or after the third stage of delivery. Choice **d** is incorrect. Abruptio placentae is a rupturing of the placenta prior to delivery.
Category: Physiological Integrity: Physiological Adaptation
Subcategory: Maternal Infant: Intrapartum

92. b. A living will is a legal document that outlines a client's wishes about life-sustaining medical treatment if the client becomes terminally ill or permanently unconscious. Choice **a** is incorrect. This statement defines a durable power of attorney. Choice **c** is incorrect. Both a living will and a durable power of attorney are considered AHCDs. Choice **d** is incorrect. A living will is considered a legal document.
Category: Safe and Effective Care Environment: Management of Care
Subcategory: Adult: Cardiovascular Disorders

93. c. Rigidity, along with irregular or erratic pulse, changes in mental status, and elevated creatinine are signs of neuroleptic malignant syndrome. Choice **a** is incorrect. Dyskinesia, although an adverse reaction to Thorazine, is not a symptom of neuroleptic malignant syndrome, which can cause irregular or erratic pulse, changes in mental status, and elevated creatinine. Choice **b** is not correct. Gait shuffling is an extrapyramidal symptom that can occur as an adverse reaction to Thorazine, but it is not a symptom of neuroleptic malignant syndrome, which can cause rigidity, irregular or erratic pulse, changes in mental status, and elevated creatinine. Choice **d** is incorrect. Toe tapping may be a symptom of hyperactivity in clients with attention deficit hyperactivity disorder (ADHD), but it is not a symptom of neuroleptic malignant syndrome.
Category: Physiological Integrity: Pharmacology and Parenteral Therapies
Subcategory: Mental Health: Medications

94. b. The client's inability to move the right leg when instructed may indicate that a hemorrhagic stroke is occurring. Immediate intervention by the nurse is required to prevent further neurologic damage. Choice **a** is incorrect. The client's headache is most likely caused by the hypertension and will require rapid nursing actions, but does not require action as urgently as the neurologic changes. Choice **c** is incorrect. The client's decreased urine output is most likely caused by the hypertension and will require rapid nursing actions, but does not require action as urgently as the neurologic changes. Choice **d** is incorrect. The client's tremors are most likely caused by the hypertension and will require rapid nursing actions, but do not require action as urgently as the neurologic changes.
Category: Physiological Integrity: Reduction of Risk
Subcategory: Adult: Cardiovascular Disorders

95. b. Acetylsalicylic acid should not be given to a child with a fever due to the risk for Reye's syndrome. Choice **a** is incorrect. Acetaminophen can be given to a child with a fever. Choice **c** is incorrect. Ibuprofen is safe to give to a child with a fever. Choice **d** is incorrect. Tepid baths can provide comfort to the child as well as assist in lowering the child's temperature.
Category: Safe and Effective Care Environment: Management of Care
Subcategory: Pediatrics: Endocrine Disorders

96. d. The recommended daily protein intake is 0.8 to 1 g/kg of body weight, which for this client is 70.4 kg × 0.8 g = 56.3 or 56 g/day. Choices **a**, **b**, and **c** are incorrect. They are not the daily minimum requirement of protein for a client who weighs 155 pounds.
Category: Health Promotion
Subcategory: Adult: Miscellaneous

97. a. Evidence of a fetus during sonogram exam is a positive sign of pregnancy. Choice **b** is incorrect. The categories for signs of pregnancy include positive, presumptive, and probable, not potential. Choice **c** is incorrect. Presumptive signs of pregnancy include breast tenderness, fatigue, morning sickness, and quickening. Choice **d** is incorrect. Probable signs of pregnancy include Goodell's sign, Hegar's sign, Chadwick's sign, and ballottement.
Category: Physiological Integrity: Basic Care and Comfort
Subcategory: Maternal Infant: Antenatal

98. b. The placement of restraints as well as skin condition, color, temperature, and sensation of restraint area must be checked at least every hour. Choice **a** is incorrect. This may provide more frequent assessment, but the standard is every hour. Choices **c** and **d** are incorrect. These intervals are too long and may increase the risk of injury.
Category: Safe and Effective Care Environment: Safety and Infection Control
Subcategory: Adult: Miscellaneous

99. a. Drooling, dystonia, and permanent gait shuffling are symptoms of tardive dyskinesia, an adverse reaction to antipsychotic medications. Choice **b** is incorrect. Pill-rolling movements, dyskinesia, and a flat affect are symptoms of drug-induced Parkinsons. Drooling, dystonia, and permanent gait shuffling are symptoms of tardive dyskinesia, an adverse reaction to antipsychotic medications. Choice **c** is incorrect. Repetitive hand motions are not a sign of tardive dyskinesia. Choice **d** is incorrect. Toe tapping and uncontrolled restlessness are symptoms of akathesia. Drooling, dystonia, and permanent gait shuffling are symptoms of tardive dyskinesia, an adverse reaction to antipsychotic medications.
Category: Physiological Integrity: Pharmacology and Parenteral Therapies
Subcategory: Mental Health: Medications

100. d. This situation indicates the client may be aspirating. The nurse's first action should be to turn off the tube feeding (4) to avoid further aspiration. The next action should be to check the client's oxygen saturation (3) because this may indicate the need for immediate respiratory suctioning and/or oxygen administration. The tube feeding residual volume should be checked next (1). This will provide data about the possible causes of aspiration. Last, the physician should be notified (2) and informed of all the assessment data the nurse has just obtained. Choices **a**, **b**, and **c** are incorrect. They are not the proper sequences of events.
Category: Physiological Integrity: Reduction of Risk
Subcategory: Adult: Neurological Disorders

101. c. Decreased protein intake should be incorporated into the child's plan of care to decrease the workload of the kidneys. Choice **a** is incorrect. The amount of carbohydrates in the diet does not need to be restricted, as the kidneys are not impacted by carbohydrates. Choice **b** is incorrect. Fluids should be increased in a child with glomerulonephritis. Choice **d** is incorrect. The child with glomerulonephritis should restrict sodium intake to decrease the workload of the kidneys.
Category: Safe and Effective Care Environment: Management of Care
Subcategory: Pediatrics: Genitourinary Disorders

102. c. The client needs to receive 1,800 mL of fluid in the first 24 hours following the burn injury. Using the Parkland formula, half of the total amount is to be infused in the first eight hours, which in this instance is 900 mL. The remaining half of the total amount is infused over the remaining 16 hours. Choices **a**, **b**, and **d** are incorrect.
Category: Physiological Integrity: Physiological Adaptation
Subcategory: Adult: Integumentary Disorders

103. c. During flexion, the fetal head bends to the chest to present the smallest diameter for delivery. Choice **a** is incorrect. During extension, upward resistance from the pelvic floor after the head has passed through the symphysis pubis causes the head to extend, which allows the occiput to emerge. Choice **b** is incorrect. During external rotation, the shoulders turn to allow for delivery of the anterior then posterior shoulder. Choice **d** is incorrect. During internal rotation, the head enters into the pelvis and then rotates 90 degrees so that the back of the neck can proceed under the symphysis pubis.
Category: Physiological Integrity: Physiological Adaptation
Subcategory: Maternal Infant: Intrapartum

104. d. Trended changes in CVP are more significant than any individual measurement. Choice **a** is incorrect. The risk of developing pulmonary edema is associated with an elevated CVP. Choice **b** is incorrect. A CVP of 15 mm Hg indicates hypervolemia, and fluid replacement would be contraindicated. Choice **c** is incorrect. The normal range for CVP is 0 to 8 mm Hg or 5 to 10 cm H_2O, depending on what type of equipment is used. A pressure greater than 6 mm Hg would fall within the normal range and therefore would not need to be reported to the physician.
Category: Physiological Integrity: Physiological Adaptation
Subcategory: Adult: Cardiovascular Disorders

105. c. The nurse should continue to monitor the client, as the lithium level is within the therapeutic range. Choice **a** is incorrect. A lithium level of 0.9 mEq/L is within the therapeutic range. Choice **b** is incorrect. The lithium level of 0.9 mEq/L is within therapeutic range, so there is no need to contact the physician at this time. Choice **d** is incorrect. Mannitol is administered to manage toxicity. A blood level of 0.9 mEq/L is not toxic; it is within the therapeutic range.
Category: Physiological Integrity: Pharmacology and Parenteral Therapies
Subcategory: Mental Health: Medications

106. d. The Allen's test is used to test blood supply to the hand, specifically, the patency of the radial and ulnar arteries. It is performed prior to radial arterial blood sampling or cannulation. Choices **a**, **b**, and **c** are incorrect. These are not the reasons why the Allen's test is performed.
Category: Physiological Integrity: Physiological Adaptation
Subcategory: Adult: Cardiovascular Disorders

107. d. Amniotic fluid that is yellow in color may indicate an infection. Choice **a** is incorrect. Amniotic fluid that is clear but with white flecks is within normal limits. Choice **b** is incorrect. Amniotic fluid that is green in color indicates fetal distress. Choice **c** is incorrect. Amniotic fluid that is the color of port wine is indicative of abruptio placentae.
Category: Safe and Effective Care Management: Safety and Infection Control
Subcategory: Maternal Infant: Intrapartum

108. b. An early symptom of type 1 diabetes is weight loss. Weight loss occurs because the body is no longer able to absorb glucose and starts to break down protein and fat for energy. Choice **a** is incorrect. The client may experience increased thirst, but will not crave fluids containing sugar. Choice **c** is incorrect. The client will experience an increased appetite; a question about anorexia is inappropriate. Choice **d** is incorrect. The client will experience polyuria, the excessive passage of urine (at least 2.5 liters per day for an adult), resulting in profuse urination and urinary frequency.
Category: Physiological Integrity: Physiological Adaptation
Subcategory: Adult: Endocrine Disorders

109. d. Eggs, milk, wheat, and soy can all be transmitted through breast milk and cause an allergic reaction in the child. Choice **a** is incorrect. Eggs, milk, and soy can all be transmitted through breast milk, as well as wheat, causing an allergic reaction in the child. Choice **b** is incorrect. Milk, wheat, and soy can all be transmitted through breast milk, as well as eggs, causing an allergic reaction in the child. Choice **c** is incorrect. Eggs, wheat, and soy can all be transmitted through breast milk, as well as milk, causing an allergic reaction in the child.
Category: Safe and Effective Care Environment: Safety and Infection Control
Subcategory: Pediatrics: Hematological/Immune System

110. d. The nurse should expect to recheck the serum potassium level during the infusion of glucose and insulin to determine the effectiveness of the therapy. Choice **a** is incorrect. The blood glucose level should be monitored during the infusion to assess for hypoglycemia or hyperglycemia; however, the serum potassium level shows the effectiveness of the therapy. Choice **b** is incorrect. The BUN and creatinine levels will not change with the administration of glucose and insulin. Choice **c** is incorrect. Changes in serum potassium level will impact the ECG and muscle strength; however, the nurse should recheck the serum potassium level to best evaluate the effects of the medications.
Category: Physiological Integrity: Physiological Adaptation
Subcategory: Adult: Renal Disorders

111. b. Delirium is precipitated by a defined event. Cognitive impairments caused by delirium are reversible once the underlying cause of the delirium is treated. Choice **a** is incorrect. The impairments caused by delirium are reversible and are precipitated by a defined event. This underlying cause of the delirium must be treated, as delirium is not a self-limiting disease. Choice **c** is incorrect. The impairments caused by delirium are not permanent, and delirium is not a self-limiting disease; the underlying cause of the delirium must be treated. Choice **d** is incorrect. The impairment caused by delirium is reversible and delirium is not a self-limiting disease; the underlying cause if the delirium must be treated.
Category: Physiological Integrity: Physiological Adaptation
Subcategory: Mental Health: Cognitive Disorders

112. c. The client's symptoms, lack of antibodies for hepatitis, and the abrupt onset of symptoms suggest toxic hepatitis can be caused by commonly used OTC drugs such as acetaminophen (Tylenol). Choice **a** is incorrect. Corticosteroid use is not associated with the symptoms listed. Choice **b** is incorrect. Jaundice is a sign of viral hepatitis, which is not indicated by the serologic testing. Choice **d** is incorrect. IV drug use is associated with viral hepatitis, which is not indicated by the serologic testing.
Category: Physiological Integrity: Physiological Adaptation
Subcategory: Adult: Gastrointestinal Disorders

113. d. Placenta previa and active genital herpes present a risk that might indicate a need for a cesarean birth. Choice **a** is incorrect. Placenta previa is a risk factor that might indicate a need for a cesarean birth but anemia is not. Choice **b** is incorrect. Active genital herpes is a risk factor that might indicate a need for a cesarean birth but anemia is not. Choice **c** is incorrect. Puerpera occurs in the postpartum period and is therefore not a risk factor that might indicate a need for a cesarean birth. Anemia is also not a risk factor.
Category: Safe and Effective Care Management: Safety and Infection Control
Subcategory: Maternal Infant: Intrapartum

114. a. The target INR for clients with atrial fibrillation is 2.0 to 3.0. The client's INR is below this range, and the dosage of warfarin should be increased. Choices **b** and **c** are incorrect. The INR level is not too high. Choice **d** is incorrect. The INR is not within the desired range.
Category: Physiological Integrity: Pharmacology and Parenteral Therapies
Subcategory: Adult: Cardiovascular Disorders

115. c. The child with sickle-cell anemia who is in a sequestration crisis experiences pooling of the blood in the spleen. Choice **a** is incorrect. Decreased red blood cell production occurs when the child with sickle-cell anemia is in an aplastic crisis. Choice **b** is incorrect. Petechia, tiny hemorrhagic spots on the skin, and bruising occur with a decrease in white blood cells in diseases such as leukemia. Choice **d** is incorrect. Swollen hands and feet occur when the child with sickle-cell anemia is in a vaso-occlusive crisis.
Category: Physiological Integrity: Physiological Adaptation
Subcategory: Pediatrics: Hematologic and Immune Disorders

116. b. Cranial nerve number nine is responsible for the pharyngeal gag reflex as well as for movement of the phonation muscles of the pharynx. It is also responsible for taste of the posterior third of the tongue and sensation from the eardrum to the ear canal. The gag reflex is tested by touching the posterior pharyngeal wall with the tongue blade and observing for gagging. Choice **a** is incorrect. Cranial nerve number six is responsible for lateral movement. Choice **c** is incorrect. Cranial nerve 12 is responsible for tongue movement. Choice **d** is incorrect. Cranial nerve five has both motor and sensory components. It is responsible for sensation in the face, scalp, oral and nasal mucosa membranes, and the cornea, and it allows chewing movement of the jaw.
Category: Health Promotion and Maintenance
Subcategory: Adult: Neurological Disorders

117. c. Timing from the beginning of one contraction to the beginning of the next measures the frequency of the contractions. Choice **a** is incorrect. Timing from the beginning of one contraction to the end of the contraction measures the duration of the contraction. Choice **b** is incorrect. From point 2 to point 5 measures the peak of one contraction to the peak of the next. Choice **d** is incorrect. Timing from the end of one contraction to the beginning of the next contraction measures the interval between contractions.
Category: Health Promotion and Maintenance
Subcategory: Maternal Infant: Intrapartum

118. a. Theophylline is a methylxanthine bronchodilator. The client needs to be taught to avoid or limit intake of foods that contain xanthine. These foods include cola, coffee, and chocolate. Choices **b**, **c**, and **d** are incorrect. These foods are not high in xanthine, which should be avoided when theophylline therapy is being administered.
Category: Physiological Integrity: Pharmacology and Parenteral Therapies
Subcategory: Adult: Respiratory Disorders

119. b. Clients with depersonalization disorders have a loss of their personal reality and feel like things are not real. Choice **a** is incorrect. Fixed, lifelike, false beliefs are associated with delusional disorders. Choice **c** is incorrect. Loss of recall of personal memories is associated with dissociative amnesia. Choice **d** is incorrect. Having two or more distinctive personalities is associated with dissociative identity disorder.
Category: Physiological Integrity: Physiological Adaptation
Subcategory: Mental Health: Dissociation Disorders

120. c. Rhinorrhea may indicate a dural tear with cerebrospinal fluid (CSF) leakage; insertion of a nasogastric tube will increase the risk for infections such as meningitis, and thus is contraindicated. Choices **a**, **b**, and **d** are incorrect. These orders are appropriate.
Category: Physiological Integrity: Physiological Adaptation
Subcategory: Adult: Neurological Disorders

121. c. Scoliosis is a lateral curvature of the spine resulting in uneven shoulders and hips and prominent scapulae. Choice **a** is incorrect. Kyphosis is an abnormal or excessive forward rounding of the upper shoulders from developmental or degenerative diseases. Choice **b** is incorrect. Lordosis is an abnormal curvature in the lumbar area of the spine resulting in a swayback posture. Choice **d** is incorrect. Scheuermann's disease is a kyphosis or forward rounding of the upper shoulders during adolescence.
Category: Physiological Integrity: Physiological Adaptation
Subcategory: Pediatrics: Musculoskeletal Disorders

122. d. The most appropriate action is to tell the client to drop and roll on the ground. This will smother the flames and put out the fire. The client's safety is the priority. Choice **a** is incorrect. This is not warranted in the instance of a fire. Choice **b** is incorrect. It is not necessary for the responding nurse to locate the fire alarm box. The other nurses who respond to the emergency can activate the fire alarm. The priority is the client's safety. Choice **c** is incorrect. Obtaining water may take too long, given where the client is in the bathroom. The priority intervention is to have the client drop to the floor and roll.
Category: Safe and Effective Care Environment: Safety and Infection Control
Subcategory: Adult: Miscellaneous

123. a. Bradycardia, a slower than normal heart rate, is a possible adverse reaction to beractant. Choice **b** is incorrect. Necrotizing enterocolitis is a complication experienced by preterm infants, but it is not an adverse reaction to beractant. Choice **c** is incorrect. Retinopathy is a complication of prematurity, but it is not an adverse reaction to beractant. Choice **d** is incorrect. An adverse reaction to beractant is bradycardia, a slower than normal heart rate, not tachycardia, a faster than normal heart rate.
Category: Physiological Integrity: Pharmacology and Parenteral Therapies
Subcategory: Maternal Infant: Intrapartum

124. c. The nurse must be aware of the physical and physiological signs of death. This is confirmed in the rigidity of the client's body and lack of change in position (2), Cheyne-Stokes respirations (3), the client's statements that he is dying (5) and is seeing family members who have already passed on (6). Findings within the normal range include blood pressure of 80/60 mm Hg (1) and extremities that are warm to the touch (4). Choices **a**, **b**, and **d** are incorrect.
Category: Psychosocial Integrity
Subcategory: Adult: Miscellaneous

125. c. Clients with an antisocial personality disorder are at risk for harming themselves or others. Choice **a** is incorrect. Delirium can be caused by substance abuse withdrawal, metabolic imbalances, or infectious diseases but is not associated with antisocial personality disorders. Choice **b** is incorrect. Hallucinations are associated with paranoid schizophrenia and substance abuse but not with antisocial personality disorder. Choice **d** is incorrect. Substance abuse can be a form of self-medication for clients with antisocial personality disorder, but the highest-priority assessment is the client's risk for harming self or others.
Category: Physiological Integrity: Physiological Adaptation
Subcategory: Mental Health: Dissociation Disorders

126. d. The Schilling's test is used to determine whether the body absorbs vitamin B_{12} normally. The client should be instructed to fast for eight hours prior to the test. No food or drink is permitted. Following the administration of the vitamin B_{12} dose, food is then delayed for three hours. Choice **a** is incorrect. The client is not required to administer a Fleets Enema prior to the procedure. Choice **b** is incorrect. It is not necessary for the client to collect his or her urine for 12 hours prior to the test. The client will be instructed to collect his or her urine after the B_{12} is administered. Choice **c** is incorrect. It is not necessary to empty the bladder prior to the test.
Category: Physiological Integrity: Physiological Adaptation
Subcategory: Adult: Hematological Disorders

127. a. Signs of ADHD include difficulty concentrating, fidgeting, and interrupting others. Choice **b** is incorrect. Hypoglycemia and hyperglycemia can cause difficulty concentrating, but fidgeting and interrupting are not usually associated with changes in blood sugars. Therefore, assessing the child's blood sugar would not be indicated. Choice **c** is incorrect. While it is appropriate for the nurse to teach the parents how to administer the child's insulin, it is important to include the child in the teaching. Choice **d** is incorrect. While written information should be given to the child and family, children with ADHD-like symptoms often have difficulty focusing on written information; therefore, it would be inappropriate to rely on written instructions as the primary teaching method.
Category: Physiological Integrity: Psychosocial Integrity
Subcategory: Pediatrics: Neurological/Cognitive Disorders

128. c. The tubing is primed with 0.9% normal saline solution. If the filter is not completely primed, debris will quickly enter the filter and the infusion will be slowed. Choice **a** is incorrect. It is neither necessary nor recommended that the blood be left at room temperature for one hour prior to the infusion. Choice **b** is incorrect. No medication should be added to the blood products. Choice **d** is incorrect. The client should have a large-bore catheter inserted for the blood transfusion.
Category: Physiological Integrity: Physiological Adaptation
Subcategory: Adult: Miscellaneous

129. d. Pregnancy during the teen years places the client at risk for preterm labor and delivery. Choice **a** is incorrect. Risk factors for anemia include multiple pregnancies, smoking, poor nutrition, and excess alcohol consumption. Choice **b** is incorrect. Risk factors for gestational diabetes include maternal age older than 35, obesity, and a family history of diabetes. Choice **c** is incorrect. Risk factors for placenta previa include advanced maternal age, previous uterine surgeries, multiple pregnancies, and multiparity.
Category: Physiological Integrity: Reduction of Risk
Subcategory: Maternal Infant: Complications

130. c. A pulsating abdominal mass is a common finding of abdominal aortic aneurysm. Choice **a** is incorrect. A boardlike, rigid abdomen may indicate internal bleeding. Choice **b** is incorrect. Knifelike pain in the back area may indicate a ruptured abdominal aneurysm. Choice **d** is incorrect. Unequal femoral pulses are not associated with an abdominal aortic aneurysm.
Category: Physiological Integrity: Physiological Adaptation
Subcategory: Adult: Cardiovascular Disorders

131. a. Athetosis refers to involuntary writhing motions in clients with cerebral palsy. Choice **b** is incorrect. Ataxia refers to uncoordinated muscle movements and a wide-based gait in clients with cerebral palsy. Choice **c** is incorrect. Hypertonia refers to rigidity or spasticity of the muscles in a client with cerebral palsy. Choice **d** is incorrect. Hypotonia refers to diminished reflexes or floppiness in a client with cerebral palsy.
Category: Physiological Integrity: Physiological Adaptation
Subcategory: Neurological/Cognitive Disorders

132. c. The symptoms suggest that the client is experiencing a pulmonary embolus. The client should be placed in the Fowler's position (semi-upright sitting position—45–60 degrees—with knees either bent or straight) to promote lung expansion and ease dyspnea. Choice **a** is incorrect. The nurse should apply oxygen via nasal cannula, but after the client is placed in a Fowler's position. Choice **b** is incorrect. The client is not choking; thus the Heimlich maneuver is not required. Choice **d** is incorrect. The Trendelenburg position (supine, or flat on the back, with the feet higher than the head by 15–30 degrees) is contraindicated in this situation.
Category: Physiological Integrity: Physiological Adaptation
Subcategory: Adult: Respiratory Disorders

133. c. The MMS is the Mini Mental Status exam, which is a set of questions designed to evaluate cognitive function. Choice **a** is incorrect. The CAGE exam is a screening tool for alcoholism that consists of four questions. Choice **b** is incorrect. The HITS exam is a screening tool for domestic violence. Choice **d** is incorrect. The PSA is a blood test that measures levels of prostate-specific antigen in the blood as a screening tool for prostate cancer.
Category: Health Promotion and Maintenance
Subcategory: Mental Health: Cognitive Disorders

134. d. A regular heart rate is calculated by multiplying the number of QRS complexes in a six-second strip by 10. In this scenario there are nine QRS complexes; thus, the heart rate is calculated at 90 bpm. This method is not accurate if the client's heart rate is irregular. Choices **a**, **b**, and **c** are incorrect. The heart rate is 90 bpm.
Category: Physiological Integrity: Physiological Adaptation
Subcategory: Adult: Cardiovascular Disorders

135. b. Harlequin changes are benign changes in the neonate's skin where one half turns dark pink or red and the other half turns pale. Choice **a** is incorrect. Acrocyanosis is cyanosis of the hands and feet in neonates. Choice **c** is incorrect. Lanugo is a fine, downy hair on the body of the neonate. Choice **d** is incorrect. Milia are small, white bumps appearing over the neonate's nose, chin, and/or cheeks.
Category: Health Promotion and Maintenance
Subcategory: Maternal Infant: Neonate Assessment

136. c. CSF is positive for glucose; thus the drainage should be tested for the presence of glucose. Choice **a** is incorrect. Testing the fluid's pH will not confirm CSF. Choices **b** and **d** are incorrect. The fluid should be tested for glucose.
Category: Physiological Integrity: Physiological Adaptation
Subcategory: Adult: Neurological Disorders

137. a. Teenagers with anorexia nervosa can have a history of binge eating and purging and/or severely restricting food intake. Choice **b** is incorrect. Teenagers with anorexia nervosa would have a BMI of less than 18.5. Choice **c** is incorrect. A symptom of anorexia nervosa is decreased sodium levels. Choice **d** is incorrect. A symptom of anorexia nervosa is absence of menorrhea.
Category: Psychosocial Integrity
Subcategory: Pediatrics

138. d. This area correctly identifies the client's bunion. A bunion results from inflammation and thickening of the first metatarsal joint of the great toe, usually with marked enlargement of the joint and the lateral displacement of the toe. Choices **a**, **b**, and **c** are incorrect. These areas do not identify a bunion.
Category: Physiological Integrity: Basic Care and Comfort
Subcategory: Adult: Musculoskeletal Disorders

139. d. The nurse should stop the oxytocin prior to administering oxygen, placing the woman in the left lateral position, or contacting the physician. Choice **a** is incorrect. Although oxygen therapy is appropriate, the nurse should first stop the oxytocin. Choice **b** is incorrect. Although the physician should be contacted, the nurse should first stop the oxytocin, place the client in the left lateral position, and administer oxygen per protocol. Choice **c** is incorrect. Although the left lateral position will promote maternal and fetal circulation and oxygenation, the nurse should first stop the oxytocin.
Category: Safe and Effective Care Management: Safety and Infection Control
Subcategory: Maternal Infant: Intrapartum

140. a. Both eyes are patched to decrease eye movement. This is done because increased eye movement can increase the amount of detachment. Choice **b** is incorrect. Patching both eyes is not done to prevent eye infections. Choice **c** is incorrect. Patching both eyes is not done to prevent photophobia. Choice **d** is incorrect. Patching both eyes is not done to prevent nystagmus.
Category: Physiological Integrity: Physiological Adaptation
Subcategory: Adult: Eye Disorders

141. d. A client with a somatic subtype of delusional disorder has an irrational belief that the body is disfigured or nonfunctional. Choice **a** is incorrect. A client with a conjugal delusional subtype has an irrational belief that a significant other has been unfaithful. Choice **b** is incorrect. A client with an erotomania delusional subtype has an irrational belief of emotional or spiritual love from a person with an elevated social status. Choice **c** is incorrect. A client with a persecutory subtype of delusional disorder has an irrational belief that there is a conspiracy against him or her.
Category: Physiological Integrity: Physiological Adaptation
Subcategory: Mental Health: Delusional Disorders

142. c. The client with liver failure will have an increased ammonia level. Ammonia is a byproduct of protein metabolism, and a diseased liver is unable to convert ammonia into urea to be excreted in the urine. Choice **a** is incorrect. The nurse would expect to see an elevated ammonia level, not decreased serum creatinine. Choice **b** is incorrect. The nurse would expect to see an elevated ammonia level, not decreased serum sodium. Choice **d** is incorrect. The nurse would expect to see an elevated ammonia level, not increased serum calcium.
Category: Physiological Integrity: Physiological Adaptation
Subcategory: Adult: Gastrointestinal Disorders

143. b. The formula for converting from Fahrenheit to Celsius is:
$C = (F - 32) \times \frac{5}{9}$.
$C = (102.5 - 32) \times \frac{5}{9} = 39.17$
Choices **a**, **c**, and **d** are incorrect.
Category: Physiological Integrity: Pharmacology and Parenteral Therapies
Subcategory: Pediatrics: Medication

144. a. A serious complication of a paracentesis is hypovolemic shock or vascular collapse. The nursing priority is monitoring the client's BP and pulse to watch for this complication. Choices **b**, **c**, and **d** are incorrect.
Category: Physiological Integrity: Physiological Adaptation
Subcategory: Adult: Gastrointestinal Disorders

145. c. In cephalohematoma, the bulge, or edema, is between the bone and periosteum and does not cross the suture lines. Choice **a** is incorrect. Anencephaly would not present as a bulge, or edema, of the soft tissues, but the head circumference might present as either equal to or smaller than the chest circumference. Choice **b** is incorrect. In caput succedaneum, the bulge, or edema, of the soft tissue of the head crosses over the suture lines (where the borders of the bony plates of the skull intersect). Choice **d** is incorrect. Hydrocephalus would present as significant swelling of the entire head, not as a bulge or swelling in a particular area of the head.
Category: Health Promotion and Maintenance
Subcategory: Maternal Infant: Neonate Assessment

146. c. The client's symptoms indicate potential respiratory distress; therefore, the nurse should prepare for intubation and mechanical ventilation. Choice **a** is incorrect. Pain medications should be administered, but the need to address the client's respiratory distress is the priority. Choice **b** is incorrect. Applying a sandbag to the flail side is contraindicated. Choice **d** is incorrect. A chest tube is not indicated for the treatment of a flail chest.
Category: Physiological Integrity: Physiological Adaptation
Subcategory: Adult: Respiratory Disorders

147. d. The correct answer is 4.5 teaspoons, determined as follows:

$$x \text{ teaspoons} = \frac{120 \text{ mg}}{1} \times \frac{15 \text{ ml}}{80 \text{ mg}} \times \frac{1 \text{ teaspoon}}{5 \text{ ml}}$$
$$= \frac{1{,}800}{400}$$
$$= 4.5 \text{ teaspoons}$$

Choices **a**, **b**, and **c** are incorrect.
Category: Physiological Integrity: Pharmacology and Parenteral Therapies
Subcategory: Pediatrics: Medication

148. b. To decrease the pressure within the compartment, the nurse should elevate the affected extremity to the level of the heart and prepare to remove/split the cast. If this intervention does not resolve the pressure, the client may require fasciotomy. Choice **a** is incorrect. Administering pain medication in this scenario is not the action to take initially. The pain from compartment syndrome does not respond well to pain medication. Choice **c** is incorrect. Intervention **b** should be implemented initially by the nurse. The physician may complete a fasciotomy if intervention **b** is unsuccessful. Choice **d** is incorrect. This position should be avoided. Placing the extremity above the level of the heart will actually increase the pressure in the compartment.
Category: Physiological Integrity: Physiological Adaptation
Subcategory: Adult: Musculoskeletal Disorders

149. a. Dependency refers to intermittent or continuous cravings for a medication or substance that leads to its repeated misuse. It would be expected that the client would no longer need to take the medication every four to six hours two months after surgery. Choice **b** is incorrect. Substance use refers to ingestion of a prescription or over-the-counter medication, alcohol, nicotine, or illicit drug. The client is using the Percocet as it was prescribed; however, it would not be expected that the client would need to take the medication every four to six hours two months after surgery. Choice **c** is incorrect. Tolerance refers to the need for increasing amounts of a medication to achieve the desired effect. Choice **d** is incorrect. Withdrawal refers to clinical symptoms produced from cessation in the user of a medication or substance.
Category: Physiological Integrity: Basic Care and Comfort
Subcategory: Mental Health: Substance Abuse

150. b. The client is at risk for bleeding. Bleeding at the site of the arterial puncture site is a serious potential problem for several hours following the completion of the procedure. Choice **a** is incorrect. The completion of a femoral arteriogram does not predispose the client to respiratory complications; general anesthetic is not used during the procedure. Choice **c** is incorrect. The client's femoral pulse should be assessed if thrombus formation at the puncture site is suspected. There is no need to assess the client's carotid pulse. Choice **d** is incorrect. The client may experience a drop in BP if bleeding is occurring. However, assessing for obvious bleeding would be the correct initial action.
Category: Physiological Integrity: Physiological Adaptation
Subcategory: Adult: Cardiovascular Disorders

151. c. Betamethasone (Celestone) is administered in two doses 24 hours apart. Choices **a** and **d** are incorrect. Betamethasone (Celestone) is administered as two IM injections 24 hours apart. Choice **b** is incorrect. Dexamethasone is administered in doses 12 hours apart, but betamethasone is administered in two doses 24 hours apart.
Category: Physiological Integrity: Pharmacology and Parenteral Therapies
Subcategory: Maternal Infant: Maternal Medication

152. a. Elevating the client's HOB to a position that will promote optimum venous outflow is the priority. The benefit of this position will be evident by a decrease in the intracranial pressure reading. Choice **b** is incorrect. Ninety degrees is too much elevation for a lethargic postoperative craniotomy with an intracranial pressure monitoring device in place. Choice **c** is incorrect. This position is contraindicated because elevating the client's legs will increase blood flow to the brain, which will further increase the client's intracranial pressure reading. Choice **d** is incorrect. The side lying position is not effective in decreasing or increasing intracranial pressure.
Category: Physiological Integrity: Physiological Adaptation
Subcategory: Adult: Neurological Disorders

153. a. The palmar grasp should disappear around three to four months of age. Choice **b** is incorrect. The plantar grasp does not disappear until eight to 10 months of age. Choice **c** is incorrect. The sucking reflex does not disappear until 10 to 12 months of age. Choice **d** is incorrect. The tonic neck reflex disappears between four and six months of age, so it is not considered an abnormal finding in a six-month-old.
Category: Physiological Integrity: Reduction of Risk
Subcategory: Pediatrics: Assessment

154. b. The nurse should have instructed the client that it is appropriate to place the casted leg on a cloth-covered pillow or blanket. These are both breathable materials that allow the cast to air-dry. No plastic should be used. Choice **a** is incorrect. Ice should be applied for 20 minutes, then removed for 20 minutes to help prevent edema of the casted extremity. Choice **c** is incorrect. Nothing should be inserted underneath the cast. Choice **d** is incorrect. Hair driers, fans, and heat lamps should not be used to help dry the cast. If used, the inside of the cast would remain damp while the outside would dry.
Category: Physiological Integrity: Reduction of Risk
Subcategory: Adult: Musculoskeletal Disorders

155. a. When administering ergot alkaloids, the nurse should closely monitor the client's blood pressure and hold the medication if the BP becomes elevated. Choice **b** is incorrect. Administration of ergot alkaloids does not cause edema as an adverse reaction. Choice **c** is incorrect. Ergot alkaloid administration may cause bradycardia, a slower than normal heart rate, not an increased heart rate (tachycardia). Choice **d** is incorrect. An adverse reaction to ergot alkaloids is respiratory depression, not an increase in the respiration rate.
Category: Physiological Integrity: Pharmacology and Parenteral Therapies
Subcategory: Maternal Infant: Maternal Medications

156. a. The nurse suspects that the client is experiencing an air embolism. An air embolism occurs frequently with central lines with sudden onset of dyspnea, hypotension, stenosis, and chest pain. The best initial nursing action is to clamp the IV line and turn the client to the left side to trap the air in the right side of the heart so it does not enter the pulmonary artery. Then call the physician and administer oxygen via nasal cannula. Choice **b** is incorrect. CPR is not necessary at this point, but should be anticipated if the client's condition deteriorates. Choice **c** is incorrect. Discontinuing and clamping the IV are the priority actions. It is not appropriate to hang another bag of IV fluids at this time. Choice **d** is incorrect. The second action the nurse should take is to notify the physician and administer oxygen via nasal cannula.
Category: Physiological Integrity: Physiological Adaptation
Subcategory: Adult: Respiratory Disorders

157. a. Disulfiram is used to assist clients to stop drinking by causing negative symptoms if alcohol is consumed while on the medication. Choice **b** is incorrect. Disulfiram is used to assist clients to stop drinking. Medications to treat anxiety include Xanax, Valium, and Ativan. Choice **c** is incorrect. Disulfiram is used to assist clients to stop drinking. Delirium is treated by first treating the underlying pathology causing the delirium. Choice **d** is incorrect. Disulfiram is used to assist clients to stop drinking. Medications used to treat depression include Wellbutrin, Celexa, Paxil, and Zoloft.
Category: Physiological Integrity: Pharmacology and Parenteral Therapies
Subcategory: Mental Health: Medications

158. b. The ventilator tubing should be checked first. Unless the client is coughing or has decreased airway compliance, or there is a hazard airway instruction, a high-pressure alarm usually indicates water collection in the ventilator tubing. Choice **a** is incorrect. The respiratory therapist does not need to be contacted. The RN should be able to check the ventilator tubing and can correct the problem. Choice **c** is incorrect. There is no indication that an arterial blood gas analysis is needed. Choice **d** is incorrect. There is no evidence of airway obstruction or excess mucus; therefore, there is no need to reposition the client to stimulate coughing.
Category: Physiological Integrity: Reduction of Risk
Subcategory: Adult: Respiratory Disorders

159. c. Pain that starts in the periumbilical area and rebound tenderness are common findings in children with appendicitis. Choice **a** is incorrect. Pain that starts in the periumbilical area is common in children with appendicitis, but the white blood cells would be expected to increase. Choice **b** is incorrect. Common assessment findings of appendicitis include increased, not decreased, white blood cells and pain in the periumbilical area, progressing to the lower right, not left, quadrant of the abdomen. Choice **d** is incorrect. While rebound tenderness is a finding associated with appendicitis, the abdominal pain is usually in the periumbilical area, progressing to the lower right quadrant of the abdomen.
Category: Safe and Effective Care Environment: Safety and Infection Control
Subcategory: Pediatrics: Gastrointestinal Disorders

160. c. The priority is for the nurse to observe the type and progression of the seizure activity. It is very important to ensure the client is safe and does not harm himself or herself during the seizure. Choice **a** is incorrect. It is important to record the length of the seizure, but this can be done only after the seizure. Choice **b** is incorrect. An aura is a warning sign that some clients experience prior to a seizure. It may include dizziness, visual or auditory disturbances, or numbness. This is not a priority assessment during the actual seizure. Choice **d** is incorrect. It is important to report what precipitated the seizure, but this is done only after the seizure.
Category: Physiological Integrity: Physiological Adaptation
Subcategory: Adult: Neurological Disorders

161. c. A client with a belief that something bad is going to happen and is unable to focus on anything else is experiencing severe anxiety. Choice **a** is incorrect. A client with mild anxiety has a worry or fear that is a part of living and does not prevent the client from focusing on other things. Choice **b** is incorrect. A client with moderate anxiety focuses on the immediate concern and is selectively inattentive to other concerns. Choice **d** is incorrect. A client experiencing panic has a sense of dread, terror, and/or impending doom and rational thought becomes lost.
Category: Physiological Integrity: Physiological Adaptation
Subcategory: Mental Health: Anxiety Disorders

162. c. The client is most likely to report a recent history of trauma, alcohol ingestion, surgical stress, or illness. All of these events are known to trigger an acute gout attack. Choice **a** is incorrect. The onset of pain, swelling, redness, and warmth is usually abrupt in nature when gout is diagnosed. Choice **b** is incorrect. The abrupt onset of symptoms of a client experiencing gout usually occurs at night with the client awakening to severe pain, swelling, redness, and warmth in the affected joint. Choice **d** is incorrect. Recent alcohol consumption or dietary changes can precipitate an event of gout.
Category: Physiological Integrity: Reduction of Risk
Subcategory: Adult: Musculoskeletal Disorders

163. a. Depressed reflexes are a sign of magnesium toxicity. Choice **b** is incorrect. Magnesium sulfate is administered to decrease the blood pressure in women with sever preeclampsia and eclampsia. Choice **c** is incorrect. Decreased, not increased, respiration is a sign of magnesium sulfate toxicity. Choice **d** is incorrect. Decreased urinary output of less than 30 ml per hour, not increased output, is a sign of magnesium sulfate toxicity.
Category: Physiological Integrity: Pharmacology and Parenteral Therapies
Subcategory: Maternal Infant: Maternal Medication

164. c. 1,000 mg:5 mL = 500 mg:x mL
$1{,}000x = 2{,}500$
$\frac{2{,}500}{1{,}000} = 2.5$ mL
Choices **a**, **b**, and **d** are incorrect.
Category: Physiological Integrity: Pharmacology and Parenteral Therapies
Subcategory: Adult: Miscellaneous

165. d. The Guthrie test is a screening test for phenylketonuria. Choice **a** is incorrect. The screening test for Down syndrome is the maternal serum alpha-fetoprotein (MSAFP) and ultrasound. Choice **b** is incorrect. Screening tests for hip dysplasia include Ortolani's and Barlow's maneuvers. Choice **c** is incorrect. Lead toxocity screening is conducted via blood analysis.
Category: Physiological Integrity: Reduction of Risk
Subcategory: Pediatrics: Endocrine Disorders

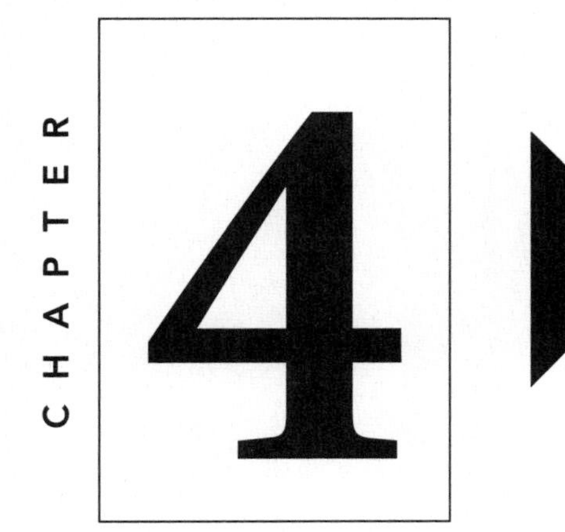

NCLEX-RN PRACTICE TEST 2

This examination has been designed to test your understanding of the content included on the National Council Licensure Examination for Registered Nurses (NCLEX-RN), which you must pass to become a registered nurse, and also to allow you to experience the format in which the exam is administered. Becoming comfortable with the examination format and logistics will help you be more relaxed when it comes to actually sitting for the test, enabling you to perform at your best.

The actual NCLEX-RN exam is computer adaptive, which means all examinees will have a different number of test questions depending on how many and what types of questions they answer correctly and how many they answer incorrectly. All test takers must answer a minimum of 75 items, and the maximum number of items that the candidate may answer is 265 during the allotted six-hour time period. This LearningExpress practice exam has 165 questions, and you should allow yourself four hours to complete it.

Then, after you have completed the exam, look at the answer key to read the rationales for both the correct and the incorrect choices, as well as the sources of the information. It is recommended that you utilize the sources to thoroughly review information that was problematic for you. Because the NCLEX-RN examination is graded on a sliding scale that is based on the difficulty of each particular exam, we are unable to predict how many correct answers would equate to an actual passing grade on this practice exam.

Completion of this examination represents the culmination of extensive test preparation. You have worked very hard to review the information from your NCLEX-RN curriculum, and now it is your time to shine. Good luck!

Practice Test 2 Answer Sheet

1. ⓐ ⓑ ⓒ ⓓ
2. ⓐ ⓑ ⓒ ⓓ
3. ⓐ ⓑ ⓒ ⓓ
4. ⓐ ⓑ ⓒ ⓓ
5. ⓐ ⓑ ⓒ ⓓ
6. ⓐ ⓑ ⓒ ⓓ
7. ⓐ ⓑ ⓒ ⓓ
8. ⓐ ⓑ ⓒ ⓓ
9. ⓐ ⓑ ⓒ ⓓ
10. ⓐ ⓑ ⓒ ⓓ
11. ⓐ ⓑ ⓒ ⓓ
12. ⓐ ⓑ ⓒ ⓓ
13. ⓐ ⓑ ⓒ ⓓ
14. ⓐ ⓑ ⓒ ⓓ
15. ⓐ ⓑ ⓒ ⓓ
16. ⓐ ⓑ ⓒ ⓓ
17. ⓐ ⓑ ⓒ ⓓ
18. ⓐ ⓑ ⓒ ⓓ
19. ⓐ ⓑ ⓒ ⓓ
20. ⓐ ⓑ ⓒ ⓓ
21. ⓐ ⓑ ⓒ ⓓ
22. ⓐ ⓑ ⓒ ⓓ
23. ⓐ ⓑ ⓒ ⓓ
24. ⓐ ⓑ ⓒ ⓓ
25. ⓐ ⓑ ⓒ ⓓ
26. ⓐ ⓑ ⓒ ⓓ
27. ⓐ ⓑ ⓒ ⓓ
28. ⓐ ⓑ ⓒ ⓓ
29. ⓐ ⓑ ⓒ ⓓ
30. ⓐ ⓑ ⓒ ⓓ
31. ⓐ ⓑ ⓒ ⓓ
32. ⓐ ⓑ ⓒ ⓓ
33. ⓐ ⓑ ⓒ ⓓ
34. ⓐ ⓑ ⓒ ⓓ
35. ⓐ ⓑ ⓒ ⓓ
36. ⓐ ⓑ ⓒ ⓓ
37. ⓐ ⓑ ⓒ ⓓ
38. ⓐ ⓑ ⓒ ⓓ
39. ⓐ ⓑ ⓒ ⓓ
40. ⓐ ⓑ ⓒ ⓓ
41. ⓐ ⓑ ⓒ ⓓ
42. ⓐ ⓑ ⓒ ⓓ
43. ⓐ ⓑ ⓒ ⓓ
44. ⓐ ⓑ ⓒ ⓓ
45. ⓐ ⓑ ⓒ ⓓ
46. ⓐ ⓑ ⓒ ⓓ
47. ⓐ ⓑ ⓒ ⓓ
48. ⓐ ⓑ ⓒ ⓓ
49. ⓐ ⓑ ⓒ ⓓ
50. ⓐ ⓑ ⓒ ⓓ
51. ⓐ ⓑ ⓒ ⓓ
52. ⓐ ⓑ ⓒ ⓓ
53. ⓐ ⓑ ⓒ ⓓ
54. ⓐ ⓑ ⓒ ⓓ
55. ⓐ ⓑ ⓒ ⓓ
56. ⓐ ⓑ ⓒ ⓓ
57. ⓐ ⓑ ⓒ ⓓ
58. ⓐ ⓑ ⓒ ⓓ
59. ⓐ ⓑ ⓒ ⓓ
60. ⓐ ⓑ ⓒ ⓓ
61. ⓐ ⓑ ⓒ ⓓ
62. ⓐ ⓑ ⓒ ⓓ
63. ⓐ ⓑ ⓒ ⓓ
64. ⓐ ⓑ ⓒ ⓓ
65. ⓐ ⓑ ⓒ ⓓ
66. ⓐ ⓑ ⓒ ⓓ
67. ⓐ ⓑ ⓒ ⓓ
68. ⓐ ⓑ ⓒ ⓓ
69. ⓐ ⓑ ⓒ ⓓ
70. ⓐ ⓑ ⓒ ⓓ
71. ⓐ ⓑ ⓒ ⓓ
72. ⓐ ⓑ ⓒ ⓓ
73. ⓐ ⓑ ⓒ ⓓ
74. ⓐ ⓑ ⓒ ⓓ
75. ⓐ ⓑ ⓒ ⓓ
76. ⓐ ⓑ ⓒ ⓓ
77. ⓐ ⓑ ⓒ ⓓ
78. ⓐ ⓑ ⓒ ⓓ
79. ⓐ ⓑ ⓒ ⓓ
80. ⓐ ⓑ ⓒ ⓓ
81. ⓐ ⓑ ⓒ ⓓ
82. ⓐ ⓑ ⓒ ⓓ
83. ⓐ ⓑ ⓒ ⓓ
84. ⓐ ⓑ ⓒ ⓓ
85. ⓐ ⓑ ⓒ ⓓ
86. ⓐ ⓑ ⓒ ⓓ
87. ⓐ ⓑ ⓒ ⓓ
88. ⓐ ⓑ ⓒ ⓓ
89. ⓐ ⓑ ⓒ ⓓ
90. ⓐ ⓑ ⓒ ⓓ
91. ⓐ ⓑ ⓒ ⓓ
92. ⓐ ⓑ ⓒ ⓓ
93. ⓐ ⓑ ⓒ ⓓ
94. ⓐ ⓑ ⓒ ⓓ
95. ⓐ ⓑ ⓒ ⓓ
96. ⓐ ⓑ ⓒ ⓓ
97. ⓐ ⓑ ⓒ ⓓ
98. ⓐ ⓑ ⓒ ⓓ
99. ⓐ ⓑ ⓒ ⓓ
100. ⓐ ⓑ ⓒ ⓓ
101. ⓐ ⓑ ⓒ ⓓ
102. ⓐ ⓑ ⓒ ⓓ
103. ⓐ ⓑ ⓒ ⓓ
104. ⓐ ⓑ ⓒ ⓓ
105. ⓐ ⓑ ⓒ ⓓ
106. ⓐ ⓑ ⓒ ⓓ
107. ⓐ ⓑ ⓒ ⓓ
108. ⓐ ⓑ ⓒ ⓓ
109. ⓐ ⓑ ⓒ ⓓ
110. ⓐ ⓑ ⓒ ⓓ
111. ⓐ ⓑ ⓒ ⓓ
112. ⓐ ⓑ ⓒ ⓓ
113. ⓐ ⓑ ⓒ ⓓ
114. ⓐ ⓑ ⓒ ⓓ
115. ⓐ ⓑ ⓒ ⓓ
116. ⓐ ⓑ ⓒ ⓓ
117. ⓐ ⓑ ⓒ ⓓ
118. ⓐ ⓑ ⓒ ⓓ
119. ⓐ ⓑ ⓒ ⓓ
120. ⓐ ⓑ ⓒ ⓓ
121. ⓐ ⓑ ⓒ ⓓ
122. ⓐ ⓑ ⓒ ⓓ
123. ⓐ ⓑ ⓒ ⓓ
124. ⓐ ⓑ ⓒ ⓓ
125. ⓐ ⓑ ⓒ ⓓ
126. ⓐ ⓑ ⓒ ⓓ
127. ⓐ ⓑ ⓒ ⓓ
128. ⓐ ⓑ ⓒ ⓓ
129. ⓐ ⓑ ⓒ ⓓ
130. ⓐ ⓑ ⓒ ⓓ
131. ⓐ ⓑ ⓒ ⓓ
132. ⓐ ⓑ ⓒ ⓓ
133. ⓐ ⓑ ⓒ ⓓ
134. ⓐ ⓑ ⓒ ⓓ
135. ⓐ ⓑ ⓒ ⓓ
136. ⓐ ⓑ ⓒ ⓓ
137. ⓐ ⓑ ⓒ ⓓ
138. ⓐ ⓑ ⓒ ⓓ
139. ⓐ ⓑ ⓒ ⓓ
140. ⓐ ⓑ ⓒ ⓓ
141. ⓐ ⓑ ⓒ ⓓ
142. ⓐ ⓑ ⓒ ⓓ
143. ⓐ ⓑ ⓒ ⓓ
144. ⓐ ⓑ ⓒ ⓓ
145. ⓐ ⓑ ⓒ ⓓ
146. ⓐ ⓑ ⓒ ⓓ
147. ⓐ ⓑ ⓒ ⓓ
148. ⓐ ⓑ ⓒ ⓓ
149. ⓐ ⓑ ⓒ ⓓ
150. ⓐ ⓑ ⓒ ⓓ
151. ⓐ ⓑ ⓒ ⓓ
152. ⓐ ⓑ ⓒ ⓓ
153. ⓐ ⓑ ⓒ ⓓ
154. ⓐ ⓑ ⓒ ⓓ
155. ⓐ ⓑ ⓒ ⓓ
156. ⓐ ⓑ ⓒ ⓓ
157. ⓐ ⓑ ⓒ ⓓ
158. ⓐ ⓑ ⓒ ⓓ
159. ⓐ ⓑ ⓒ ⓓ
160. ⓐ ⓑ ⓒ ⓓ
161. ⓐ ⓑ ⓒ ⓓ
162. ⓐ ⓑ ⓒ ⓓ
163. ⓐ ⓑ ⓒ ⓓ
164. ⓐ ⓑ ⓒ ⓓ
165. ⓐ ⓑ ⓒ ⓓ

Questions

1. A client is prescribed lisinopril (Zestril) for the treatment of hypertension. The client asks the nurse about possible side effects of the medication. The nurse will relay that which of the following are common adverse effects of angiotensin-converting enzyme (ACE) inhibitors? Select all that apply.

1. constipation
2. dizziness
3. headache
4. hyperglycemia
5. hypotension
6. impotence

a. 1, 4, 6
b. 2, 3, 5
c. 1, 3, 4, 6
d. 2, 4, 5, 6

2. A woman comes to the labor and delivery triage area stating that she is in labor. The nurse determines that the client is in true labor due to which of the following?

a. cervical dilation of 4 cm
b. contractions that decrease when sitting
c. contractions that decrease with ambulation
d. lightening

3. A graduate nurse is completing a critical-care nursing course. The nurse will identify which of the following as the QRS complex?

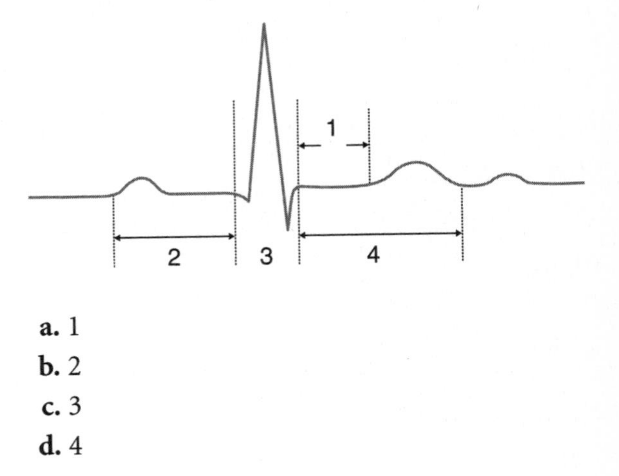

a. 1
b. 2
c. 3
d. 4

4. A nurse is preparing to administer an intramuscular (IM) injection to a four-year-old girl. Where should the nurse plan to administer the injection?

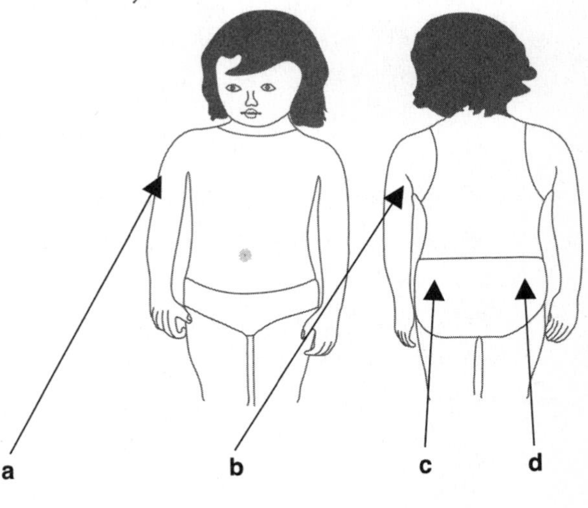

5. A client is being treated in a medical-surgical unit following an ileostomy placement. The nurse is teaching the client about diet following the surgery. It is important for the nurse to include which of the following in the dietary instructions?

a. "Chewing your food thoroughly will aid in digestion."
b. "Eating six small meals a day will prevent abdominal distention."
c. "It is necessary to limit your fluid intake to 100 mL per day."
d. "You can eat anything you want; monitoring your diet is not necessary."

6. A young male client is admitted to the hospital with Hodgkin's disease. The client has been unresponsive to multiple therapeutic interventions. Death appears imminent. A priority goal in the treatment of this client is which of the following?

a. Reduce the client's fear of more aggressive treatment.
b. Reduce the client's fear of pain.
c. Reduce the client's feelings of fear.
d. Reduce the client's feelings of isolation.

7. A nurse is completing the medication-reconciliation list on a client admitted with pneumonia. One of the medications is Remeron. The nurse knows that this medication is used in clients with which of the following?

a. anxiety
b. bipolar disorder
c. depression
d. sleep disorders

8. A nurse is preparing to administer prostaglandin E to a pregnant woman who is at 40 weeks gestation. Which intervention should the nurse implement first?

a. Assess for patency of IV access.
b. Have the client void prior to initiating the therapy.
c. Monitor for stomach cramping.
d. Position the client so that she is lying on her left side.

9. A client diagnosed with renal failure has just started peritoneal dialysis treatments. During the infusion of the dialysate, the client begins to complain of abdominal pain. Which of the following actions is most appropriate for the nurse to complete?

a. Decrease the amount of dialysate solution being infused.
b. Explain to the client that the pain will decrease after more exchanges.
c. Slow down with the infusion rate.
d. Stop the dialysis session immediately.

10. A nurse is assessing an infant for hip dysplasia. The maneuver pictured is called what?

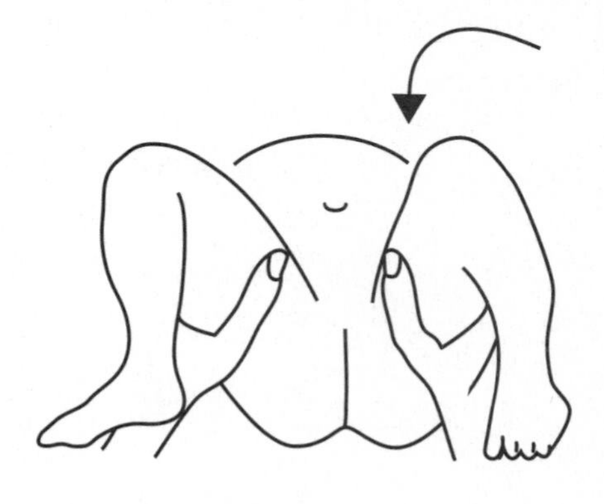

a. Barlow's maneuver
b. Chadwick's sign
c. Hegar's sign
d. Ortolani's maneuver

11. A nurse in the neonatal intensive care unit (NICU) is planning to administer the prescribed lung surfactant, beractant, to a neonate via endotracheal tube. She knows that beractant is administered to preterm infants for prevention and treatment of
a. asthma.
b. neonatal croup.
c. respiratory distress syndrome.
d. sudden infant death syndrome.

12. A nurse is caring for a client with metastatic breast cancer on the oncology unit. The client is to receive tamoxifen (Nolvadex). The nurse must specifically monitor which of the following laboratory values while the client is taking this medication?
a. calcium level
b. glucose level
c. potassium level
d. prothrombin time

13. A client is admitted to the hospital to rule out colon cancer. A diagnostic study of the colon is ordered. The nurse teaches the client how to self-administer a prepackaged enema. Which of the following statements by the client indicates effective teaching?
a. "I will administer the enema while lying on my back with both knees flexed."
b. "I will administer the enema while lying on my left side with my right knee flexed."
c. "I will administer the enema while lying on my right side with my left knee flexed."
d. "I will administer the enema while sitting on the bathroom toilet."

14. A nurse suspects benzodiazepine toxicity in a client taking Tranxene. Expected assessment findings would include which of the following? Select all that apply.
1. hyperactivity
2. confusion
3. increased reflexes
4. somnolence

a. 1, 4
b. 2, 3
c. 2, 4
d. 1, 3

15. A client at 38 weeks gestation comes into the labor and delivery triage area. The client has been experiencing contractions that are irregular in frequency, are localized in the abdomen, and decrease when the client ambulates. The client has no cervical changes. The nurse should
a. instruct the client to ambulate in the halls.
b. instruct the client to return home.
c. prepare the client for admission.
d. prepare the client for cesarean section.

16. A client is being discharged from a cardiac step-down unit following the insertion of a permanent pacemaker in the upper left chest area. Upon discharge, the nurse should include which of the following instructions? Select all that apply.
1. Avoid air travel because of security alarms.
2. Avoid lifting objects heavier than three pounds.
3. A microwave cannot be used.
4. Immobilize the affected arm for four to six weeks.
5. Take and record your daily pulse rate.

a. 1, 3, 4
b. 3, 4, 5
c. 1, 2
d. 2, 5

17. A nurse is caring for a child with tetralogy of Fallot. The nurse knows that this disorder involves which four of the following defects? Select all that apply.

1. left ventricular hypertrophy
2. overriding aorta
3. patent ductus arteriosus
4. pulmonary stenosis
5. right ventricular hypertrophy
6. ventral septal defect

a. 1, 2, 3, 4
b. 2, 4, 5, 6
c. 3, 4, 5, 6
d. 1, 3, 5, 6

18. A nurse is working in the child development unit. In which child should the nurse consider that a developmental delay exists?

a. a two-month-old who is unable to transfer objects from hand to hand
b. a six-month-old who is unable to play peekaboo
c. a 14-month-old who is unable to pull up into a standing position
d. a 16-month-old who is unable to use a fork

19. A client is being treated in the hospital for chronic renal failure. The client has been placed on a 500 mL per day fluid restriction. During the nurse's late evening assessment, the client is requesting additional fluids. Which of the following is the most appropriate nursing intervention?

a. Explain to the client the importance of the fluid restriction.
b. Disregard the client's request.
c. Give the client a piece of hard candy.
d. Tell the client that you will speak to the physician about the request.

20. A nurse is working on a mental health unit with a client. The nurse is trying to help the client understand that his frequent loud, angry outbursts are disruptive and cause others to avoid him. This is an example of which type of therapy?

a. behavioral
b. cognitive
c. crisis
d. milieu

21. A nurse has just completed a neurological exam on a client. The client is exhibiting decerebrate posturing. Which of the following correctly describes the decerebrate posturing?

a. back arched, rigid extension of all four extremities
b. back hunched over, rigid flexion of all four extremities with supination of arms and palmar flexion of the feet
c. internal rotation and abduction of arms with flexion of the elbows, wrists, and fingers
d. supination of the arms with dorsal flexion of the feet

22. A nurse is assessing the growth and height of a five-year-old boy. The boy's height is 115 cm and his weight is 15 kg. After documenting the child's growth on the following growth chart, the nurse should include which of the following interventions into the child's plan of care?

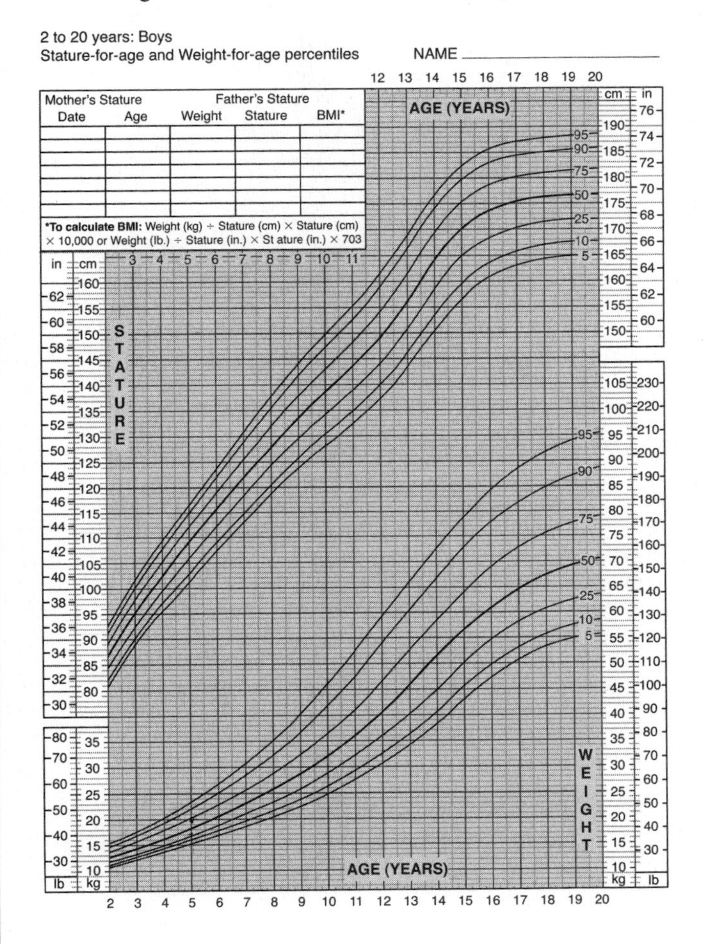

a. increased nutritious snacks
b. increased physical activity
c. decreased caloric intake
d. television viewing limits

23. A nurse is caring for clients in a postpartum unit. Which client should the nurse attend to first?

a. the breast-feeding client with sore nipples
b. the client with a first-degree perineal laceration
c. the client with lochia rubra
d. the client with a soft, boggy uterus

24. A graduate nurse is participating in a basic health-assessment course. The nurse correctly identifies Erb's point at which location?

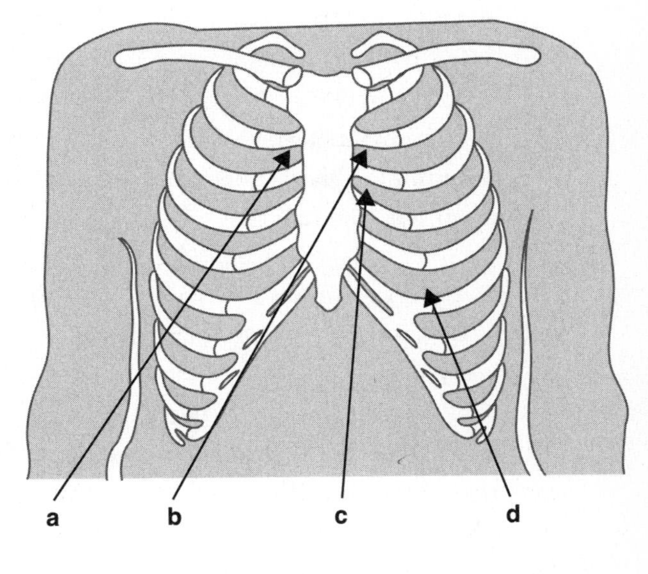

25. A client is admitted to the ICU following a mitral valve replacement. The client has persistent bleeding from the sternal incision during the early postoperative period. It is imperative that the nurse complete which of the following? Select all that apply.

1. Administer warfarin (Coumadin).
2. Begin intravenous dopamine (Inotropin) for a systolic BP ≤ 100.
3. Confirm the availability of blood products.
4. Evaluate postoperative laboratory reports, including complete blood count (CBC), international normalized ratio (INR), partial thromboplastin time (PTT), and platelet levels.
5. Monitor the mediastinal chest-tube drainage.

a. 1, 3
b. 2, 5
c. 1, 2, 4
d. 3, 4, 5

26. A nurse is caring for a client and notes that the parenteral nutrition (PN) bag is empty. Which of the following solutions should the nurse hang until another PN solution is mixed and delivered to the nursing unit?
a. 5% dextrose in Ringer's lactate
b. 5% dextrose in water
c. 5% dextrose in 0.9% sodium chloride
d. 10% dextrose in water

27. A nurse's goal with group therapy is to
a. assess family functioning.
b. identify immediate coping patterns.
c. replace negative attitudes and behaviors.
d. resolve emotional and self-esteem issues.

28. A child is admitted to the pediatric unit due to patent ductus arteriosus. Where on the picture is this defect located?

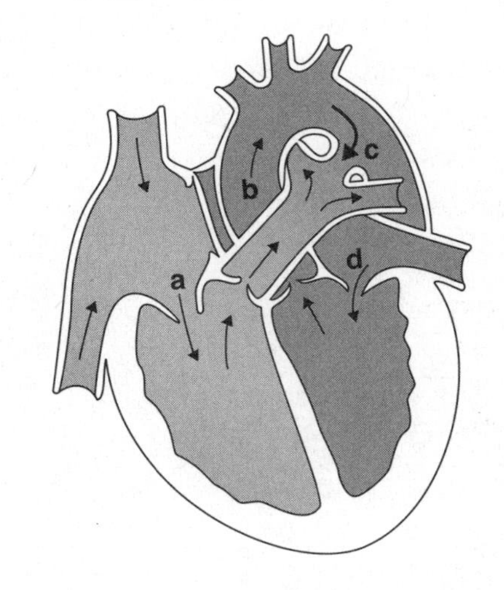

29. A nurse is assessing a client for probable signs of pregnancy during the first prenatal visit. Which of the following signs would the nurse expect to find?
a. breast tenderness
b. missed period
c. Chadwick's sign
d. fetal heartbeat

30. A nurse is caring for a client recently diagnosed with glaucoma. The client is prescribed miotic medication. When teaching the client about medication effects, the nurse will inform the client that this medication will produce which of the following effects?
a. dilated pupil to reduce intraocular pressure
b. interrupted drainage of aqueous humor from the eye
c. lowered intraocular pressure and enhanced blood flow to the retina
d. reshaped lines of the eye to eliminate blurred vision

31. A nurse has received a nursing report. Which of the following client data is assessed as the highest priority?
a. hemoglobin level: 14.6 gm/dL
b. pulse oximetry reading: 85%
c. urine output: 250 mL/8 hours
d. serum potassium level: 3.8 mEq/L

32. A nurse is caring for a client who obsessively washes his hands. The nurse should
a. focus the client's attention on the behavior.
b. ignore the compulsive behavior.
c. prevent the client from washing his hands.
d. set defined times for hand washing.

33. A client is being educated about the complications of peritoneal dialysis. Which of the following should the nurse teach the client about preventing peritonitis? Select all that apply.
1. Antibiotics may be added to the dialysate to treat peritonitis.
2. Broad-spectrum antibiotics can be administered to prevent infection.
3. Peritonitis is characterized by cloudy dialysate drainage and abdominal pain.
4. Peritonitis is the most serious and common complication of peritoneal dialysis.
5. Utilizing clean technique is permissible for the prevention of peritonitis.

a. 1, 5
b. 2, 4
c. 1, 2, 3, 4
d. 1, 2, 3, 4, 5

34. A client is in her second trimester of pregnancy. She tells the nurse that she is always thirsty and that she has been voiding more than usual. Based on this information, the nurse should check for
a. edema.
b. glycosuria.
c. proteinuria.
d. tinnitus.

35. A nurse is providing discharge instructions to the parents of a 10-year-old child with rheumatic heart disease. The nurse determines that the parents have understood the discharge instructions when the mother states,
a. "I hold digoxin if the heart rate is greater than 60 bpm."
b. "I give the antibiotic once a month."
c. "I should not give my child Tylenol."
d. "I should not give my child aspirin."

36. A male client receives hemodialysis treatments three times a week. The home health nurse is assessing the client's ability to self-monitor between the dialysis treatments. The nurse determines the client is fully informed when he states that he records which of the following on a daily basis?
a. blood urea nitrogen (BUN) and creatinine levels
b. daily living activities and periods of weakness
c. intake and output and weight
d. respiratory and heart rates

37. A client who is 32 weeks pregnant and experiencing a healthy pregnancy is in the office for a routine prenatal visit. She asks when she should return for her next prenatal visit. The nurse should schedule the client's next prenatal visit for when?
a. in one week
b. in two weeks
c. in three weeks
d. in four weeks

38. A client with the following cardiac telemetry reading is being discharged home after an unsuccessful cardioversion attempt.

The nurse understands the client will be instructed to take which of the following medications in order to prevent thromboembolic complications of this dysrhythmia?

a. aspirin (acetylsalicylic acid)
b. Coumadin (warfarin sodium)
c. heparin
d. Ticlid (ticlopidine)

39. A nurse is caring for a client with Alzheimer's disease who frequently repeats statements and questions. The nurse knows that the part of the client's brain that is being affected by the disease is which of the following areas?

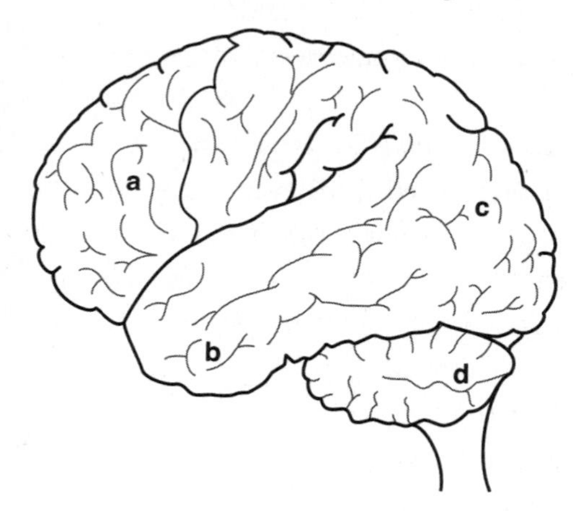

40. A nurse is completing a physical assessment on a healthy five-year-old during a well child visit. Which of the following would the nurse expect to find during the respiratory assessment? Select all that apply.

1. abdominal breathing
2. anterior-to-posterior ratio 1:1
3. hyperresonant lung sounds
4. respiratory rate of 14 breaths per minute

a. 1, 2
b. 1, 3
c. 2, 3
d. 2, 4

41. A nurse is caring for a client diagnosed with ulcerative colitis. The nurse recognizes that an expected outcome of the medical regimen has been achieved when which of the following occurs?

a. The client verbalizes acceptance of an ileostomy.
b. The client's episodes of constipation decrease.
c. The client maintains an ideal body weight.
d. The client states the importance of decreasing fluid intake.

42. A nurse is caring for a client diagnosed with diabetes. The nurse is assessing the client for common complications related to this disorder. In doing so, the nurse should include an examination of which of the following?

a. abdomen
b. eyes
c. lymph glands
d. pharynx

43. A client has been seen and treated for gastrointestinal reflux in the emergency department. Which of the following client statements indicates to the nurse that the client understands how to prevent reflux?

a. "It is important for me to lie down and rest for 35 minutes after meals."
b. "I will eat smaller meals more frequently throughout the day."
c. "I will increase my fluids with meals to help with digestion."
d. "I will sleep on my left side to empty my stomach contents."

44. A nurse is working with a client who has a history of early Alzheimer's disease. The nurse wants the client to take her medications and then get dressed. The nurse should tell the client,

a. "Don't get dressed until you take your medications."
b. "Take your medications and then get dressed."
c. "Get dressed." (This is said after the client has taken her medications.)
d. "Take your medications." (This is said after the client has eaten breakfast.)

45. A nurse is providing nutritional counseling for a client at 12 weeks gestation. The nurse should teach the client to do which of the following?

a. Avoid undercooked eggs and meats.
b. Decrease sodium intake.
c. Limit caffeine intake to 800 mg per day.
d. Limit folic-acid-fortified breads and cereals.

46. A client is admitted to the emergency department with second-degree burns to the anterior portion of the right leg and to the anterior and posterior portions of the right arm. Based on the rule of nines, the triage nurse will document what percentage of total body surface area (TBSA) burned?

a. 18%
b. 27%
c. 36%
d. 45%

47. A nurse is caring for a client who has been ordered a dose of iron by the parenteral route. The nurse is aware that which of the following actions should be taken to decrease pain at the injection site?

a. changing the needle used to draw up the medication prior to injection to prevent bruising at the site
b. gently massaging the injection site to increase absorption of the prescribed medication
c. using a Z-track method for intramuscular injection of the prescribed medication
d. utilizing an air lock when drawing up the prescribed medication

48. A charge nurse on a medical-surgical unit is preparing to make morning assignments for the nursing staff. Which of the following nursing activities may be delegated to the licensed practical nurse or licensed vocational nurse (LPN/LVN)? Select all that apply.

1. endotracheal suctioning
2. client admission assessments
3. intravenous medication administration
4. intramuscular medication administration
5. subcutaneous medication administration
6. urinary catheterization

a. 1, 2, 3, 5
b. 1, 4, 5, 6
c. 2, 4
d. 3, 5

49. A father brings his two-month-old child to the clinic for a well child exam. The nurse knows that according to Centers for Disease Control and Prevention (CDC) immunization recommendations, the child will be due for which of the following vaccinations?
a. DTaP (diphtheria, tetanus, pertussis)
b. influenza
c. MMR (measles, mumps, rubella)
d. varicella

50. A client diagnosed with post-traumatic stress disorder is having difficulty falling asleep at night. To promote sleeping, the nurse should
a. administer amitriptyline.
b. have the client watch television.
c. help the client establish a routine.
d. sit in the room with the client.

51. A nurse is admitting a client who is 28 weeks pregnant and is experiencing uterine contractions every 10 minutes that are not relieved by changing position. Her cervix is dilated to 4 cm and her blood pressure is 122/72 mm Hg. The client's pulse is 78 beats per minutes and her respirations are 20 breaths per minute. Based on this information, the client might be experiencing which complication of pregnancy?
a. cervical incompetence
b. placenta previa
c. preeclampsia
d. preterm labor

52. A graduate nurse needs to administer potassium chloride intravenously to a client with hypokalemia. The nursing preceptor determines that the graduate nurse is unprepared for this procedure if the graduate states that which of the following is part of the plan for the preparation and administration of potassium chloride intravenously?
a. diluting the potassium chloride in the appropriate amount of normal saline
b. monitoring the client's urine output during the infusion process
c. obtaining a controlled electronic IV pump for infusion
d. preparing the potassium chloride for intravenous bolus injection

53. A 37-year-old client, who has four children and is a waitress by occupation, is seen in the outpatient clinic for a routine checkup. The nurse caring for this client realizes she is at risk for developing which of the following peripheral vascular disorders?
a. acute arterial embolism
b. arterial insufficiency
c. thrombophlebitis
d. varicose veins

54. When communicating with a client who speaks a different language, the nurse is aware that it is the best practice to complete which of the following?

a. Arrange for an interpreter when communicating with the client.
b. Speak loudly and clearly when communicating with the client.
c. Speak to the client only when family is present to enhance communication.
d. Stand close to the client and speak loudly during interactions.

55. A client with premature rupture of the membranes is in labor. Suddenly, the client experiences an acute onset of respiratory distress, chest pain, and hypotension. The fetal monitor indicates a decrease in the fetal heart rate. The nurse should immediately place the client in which of the following positions?

a. left lateral
b. right lateral
c. semi-Fowler's
d. Trendelenburg

56. A client presents to the emergency room with complaints of chest pain that began five hours ago. A troponin-T blood-serum analysis is obtained, the results of which reveal a level of 0.7 ng/mL. The nurse recognizes that this result indicates which of the following?

a. a level that is in the normal range
b. a level that indicates the presence of angina
c. a level that indicates myocardial infarction
d. a level that indicates possible gastritis

57. A nurse is providing education to the parents of an 11-year-old girl regarding the CDC recommendations for immunizations for 11-year-old girls. The nurse realizes additional education is needed when the mother states that her daughter needs which vaccination?

a. HPV (human papillomavirus)
b. inactivated polio virus
c. influenza
d. MCV4 (meningococcal conjugate vaccine)

58. An elderly woman is brought to the emergency department by her son for treatment of a fractured left arm. On assessment, the nurse notes old and new areas of ecchymosis on the client's legs and chest. The nurse asks the client how she sustained these injuries. The client, although reluctant, tells the nurse in confidence that her live-in boyfriend frequently hits her when the house is not clean. Which of the following is the most appropriate nursing response?

a. "Do you have any friends that you can stay with until you get these issues resolved with your boyfriend?"
b. "Let's talk about specific ways you can manage your time to help prevent this from happening again."
c. "This is a legal issue, and it's important for you to recognize that I will have to report it to the proper authorities."
d. "This is unacceptable behavior by your boyfriend; I will need to speak to him and your son immediately about the situation."

59. For a client with bulimia nervosa, the nurse's plan of care should include which of the following? Select all that apply.
1. providing calorie-dense foods
2. establishing a client food contract
3. staying with the client two hours after she eats
4. limiting time in the bathroom

a. 1, 2
b. 2, 3
c. 3, 4
d. 1, 4

60. A nurse is reviewing laboratory results for a client for whom she is assigned care. The client's potassium level is recorded at 3.1 mEq/L. The nurse recognizes this would explain the presence of which of the following on the electrocardiogram?
a. absent P-waves
b. elevated ST segments
c. elevated T-waves
d. U-waves

61. A nurse is caring for a client in the neurological intensive care unit. The client has a history of a seizure disorder and is receiving dilantin (Phenytoin). Which of the following is a therapeutic serum dilantin level for a client with a history of seizures?
a. 9 μg/mL
b. 16 μg/mL
c. 28 μg/mL
d. 37 μg/mL

62. A newborn infant was circumcised earlier in the day. The manager of the nurse caring for the infant recognizes that the nurse understands the infant's nursing care needs when the manager observes the nurse performing which of the following interventions?
a. assessing the circumcision site for signs of bleeding and/or infection
b. cleansing the circumcision site with a baby wipe
c. placing a petroleum gauze around the circumcision site and then placing the infant in the radiant warmer
d. securing the infant's diaper tightly to apply pressure to the circumcision site

63. A client is admitted to the medical-surgical unit with a diagnosis of diabetes mellitus. The client received NPH insulin at 7 a.m. The nurse must carefully monitor the client for hypoglycemia between which of the following time periods?
a. 9 a.m.–11 a.m.
b. 1 p.m.–7 p.m.
c. 7 p.m.–11 p.m.
d. midnight–6 a.m.

64. The hospital's standing orders for newborns include eye prophylaxis medication to be administered within the first hour of birth. The nurse understands that this is to protect the infant's eyes from which of the following infections?
a. candidiasis
b. genital herpes
c. gonorrhea
d. B strep

65. A nurse is preparing to change the parenteral nutrition (PN) solution bag and tubing. The client's central venous line is located in the right subclavian vein. The nurse will ask the client to take which of the following actions during the tubing change?

a. Breathe as normally as possible.
b. Exhale evenly and slowly.
c. Take a deep breath, hold it, and bear down.
d. Turn the head to the right side.

66. A nurse in a pediatric unit is caring for a child with congestive heart failure. The nurse should perform which of the following interventions?

a. administer morphine sulfate
b. lower the head of the bed
c. offer small meals frequently
d. provide a stimulating environment

67. A client is complaining of chest pain. The graduate nurse is performing a 12-lead electrocardiogram (ECG). Identify the area where lead V6 should be placed.

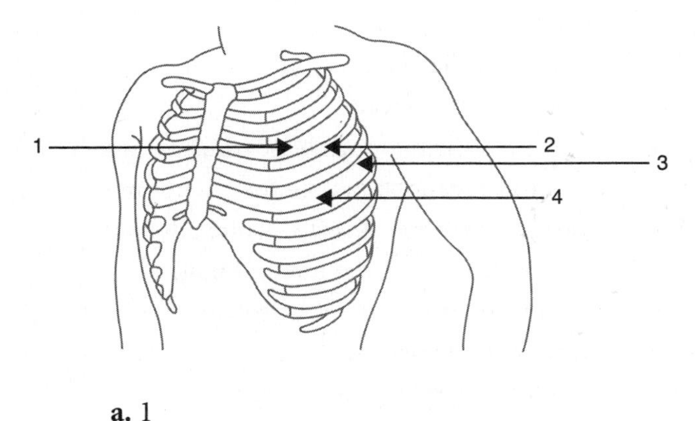

a. 1
b. 2
c. 3
d. 4

68. A nurse is caring for a client in the manic phase of bipolar disorder. The nurse's plan of care should include interventions that address which of the following symptoms?

a. impulsiveness
b. feelings of hopelessness
c. suicidal thoughts
d. anxiety

69. A client is admitted to the emergency department complaining of burning on urination. Upon assessment, it is apparent that the client has a low-grade fever. The physical examination also reveals right-sided costovertebral tenderness. Identify the area the nurse percussed to elicit this sign.

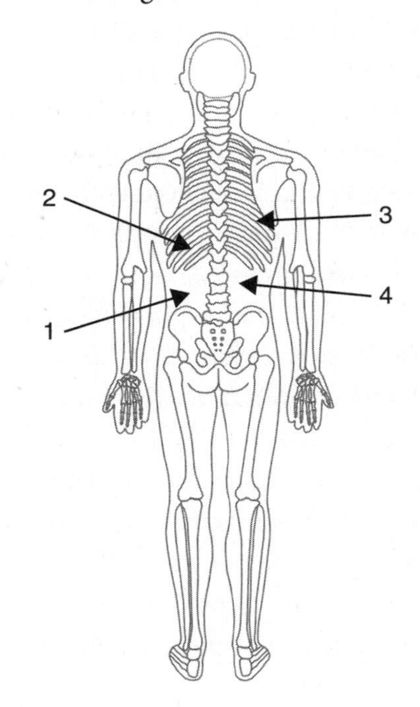

a. 1
b. 2
c. 3
d. 4

70. A nurse on orientation is completing umbilical-cord care on a newborn who is six hours old. The nurse is preparing to unclamp the cord. Which action by the unit nursing educator observing the nurse is best?

a. Distract the newborn with a brightly colored object.
b. Instruct the nurse that the cord should shrivel and fall off within 7 to 10 days.
c. Encourage the nurse to unclamp the cord.
d. Stop the nurse from unclamping the cord.

71. A nurse is caring for a client with complications related to rheumatoid arthritis. Which of the following statements might indicate a violation of client confidentiality?

a. The nurse discussed the client's condition and diagnosis with a family friend over the telephone.
b. The nurse discussed the client's condition and diagnosis with another nurse at shift report.
c. The nurse discussed the client's medication therapy with the hospital pharmacist.
d. The nurse discussed the client's medication therapy with the physician.

72. A client in the cardiovascular step-down unit is having a chest tube removed following open heart surgery. During the chest tube removal, the nurse instructs the client to complete which of the following activities?

a. Exhale slowly.
b. Inhale and exhale quickly.
c. Perform the Valsalva maneuver.
d. Stay very still during the procedure.

73. A nurse is instructing a client diagnosed with pneumonia on how to use an incentive spirometer properly. The nurse should instruct the client to implement the following steps. Place the following steps in order from first to last.

1. The client should exhale fully.
2. The client should inhale on the mouthpiece and hold the breath for three seconds.
3. The client should passively exhale.
4. The client should take a deep breath and cough.

a. 1, 2, 3, 4
b. 2, 1, 4, 3
c. 3, 2, 1, 4
d. 4, 1, 2, 3

74. A nurse is caring for a child with aortic stenosis. Which of the following would the nurse NOT expect to find upon assessment?

a. congestive cough
b. cyanosis
c. fatigue
d. tachycardia

75. A nurse is caring for a client admitted with severe depression who has lost 25 pounds in the past three months. To ensure adequate nutritional intake, the nurse should

a. allow the client to select meals.
b. attractively present large meals.
c. offer finger foods frequently.
d. provide calorie-dense foods.

76. A nurse is caring for a client with an infant daughter who is seven hours old. The client is wondering why the infant has downy hair on her chest and face. Which of the following is the best response by the nurse?

a. "That is unusual; I have not seen this before."
b. "That is lanugo and it will disappear on its own."
c. "That is milia and it will disappear on its own."
d. "That is lanugo and it will need to be surgically removed."

77. A client in the ICU is diagnosed with a myocardial infarction. The client develops cardiogenic shock. Which of the following characteristic signs should the nurse expect to observe in this client?

a. bradycardia
b. elevated blood pressure
c. fever
d. oliguria

78. A nurse is administering Pitocin to a client to induce labor. The nurse realizes that because of this, the client will need close monitoring in the postpartum period for

a. hemorrhage.
b. hyperglycemia.
c. hypoglycemia.
d. orthostatic hypotension.

79. A client is being treated in the ICU for a hypertensive crisis. The nurse is to administer sodium nitroprusside (Nipride). The medication comes in a dilution of 50 mg/250 mL. How many micrograms of Nipride are in each milliliter?

a. 10 mcg
b. 20 mcg
c. 100 mcg
d. 200 mcg

80. A client who is eight weeks pregnant is experiencing morning sickness. The nurse instructs the patient to

a. eat dry crackers prior to getting out of bed in the morning.
b. eat three large meals per day.
c. increase the amount of fatty foods in her diet.
d. increase the amount of fluids she has with her meals.

81. A client is admitted to the neurological ICU following a craniotomy. The nurse and the medical staff have established a goal to maintain the client's intracranial pressure (ICP) within normal range. Which of the following should the nurse do? Select all that apply.

1. Assure the head of the bed is elevated 15 to 30 degrees.
2. Encourage the client to cough and breathe deeply often.
3. Monitor the client's neurological status using the Glasgow Coma Scale (GCS).
4. Notify the healthcare provider if the ICP is greater than 20 mm Hg.
5. Stimulate the client with the use of active range-of-motion exercises.

a. 2, 5
b. 1, 3, 4
c. 3, 4, 5
d. 2, 3, 4, 5

82. A nurse and graduate nurse are caring for a client diagnosed with Parkinson's disease. The graduate nurse asks the nurse what the initial sign of Parkinson's disease is. Which of the following is a correct response by the nurse?

a. akinesia
b. bradykinesia
c. rigidity
d. tremors

83. A nurse is admitting a child diagnosed with rheumatic fever to the pediatric unit. The nurse should assess for which of the following?
a. decreased sedimentation rate
b. history of viral throat infection
c. pain in the joints
d. inspiratory pain

84. A nurse is caring for a client with pulmonary congestion. The physician orders chest physiotherapy. When should the nurse plan to perform chest physiotherapy?
a. after meals
b. before meals
c. when the client has time
d. when the nurse has time

85. A client diagnosed with depression is taking the medication Celexa. The client is beginning to experience increased energy and improved affect. When planning the client's care, the nurse's priority is to
a. allow the client to verbalize feelings.
b. assess for thoughts of suicide.
c. ensure adequate nutritional intake.
d. monitor the client's blood pressure.

86. A client is breast-feeding her two-week-old infant. The client complains of sore, cracked nipples. The nurse realizes that cracked nipples
a. are a normal occurrence for clients who are breast-feeding.
b. are often caused by the infant's latching on incorrectly.
c. can be prevented by having the client guide only the nipple into the infant's mouth.
d. can be prevented by washing the nipples after each feeding with soap and water.

87. A nurse is caring for a client with a head injury. Upon assessment, the nurse finds the client in the position pictured.

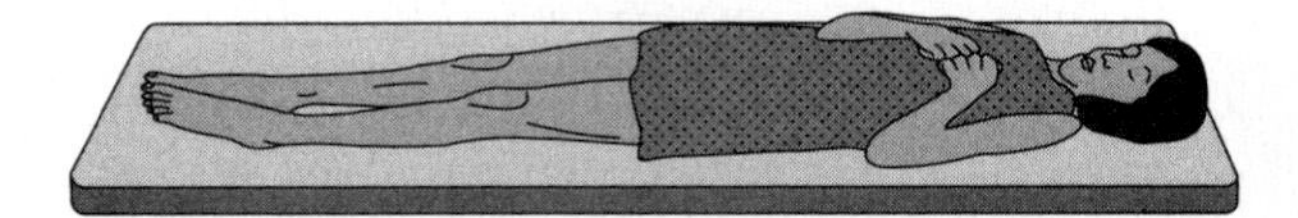

The nurse will correctly document this as which of the following?
a. decerebrate
b. decorticate
c. opisthotonus
d. prone

88. A nurse is caring for a client who is diagnosed with gout. Which of the following foods should the nurse instruct the client NOT to eat? Select all that apply.
1. chocolate
2. cod
3. eggs
4. green, leafy vegetables
5. liver
6. sardines

a. 1, 3, 4
b. 2, 5, 6
c. 2, 3, 4, 5
d. 1, 2, 3, 5

89. The Apgar score of a neonate at one minute after birth is 6. The nurse should prepare to perform which nursing intervention?
a. Administer oxygen to the infant.
b. Begin resuscitation measures.
c. Give the infant its first bath.
d. Place the infant on the mother's chest to promote bonding.

90. A mother asks a nurse how she should take the temperature of her three-year-old daughter. Which of the following should be the nurse's response? Select all that apply.

1. axillary
2. oral
3. tympanic
4. rectal

a. 1, 2
b. 1, 3
c. 1, 4
d. 2, 4

91. A nurse is completing a dressing change for a client in the burn unit. The client is prescribed mafenide acetate (Sulfamylon). While applying the medication to the burned area, the client complains of local discomfort and burning. Which of the following is the most appropriate action for the nurse to take in this situation?

a. Apply a thinner layer of the medication.
b. Discontinue using the medication.
c. Notify the healthcare provider.
d. Tell the client this is normal.

92. A nurse is caring for a client experiencing acute respiratory failure. The nurse will focus on resolving which of the following?

a. hypoventilation, hypoxemia, and hypercapnia
b. hyperoxemia, hypocapnia, and hyperventilation
c. hyperventilation, hypertension, and hypocapnia
d. hypotension, hyperoxemia, and hypercapnia

93. A 24-year-old female client presents to the community medical clinic complaining of a 20-pound weight loss over the prior month even though she has felt "famished" and hasn't changed her activity level. After further assessment, the nurse learns the client has a diagnosis of Graves' disease. Which other signs and symptoms support the diagnosis of Graves' disease? Select all that apply.

1. bounding, rapid pulses
2. bradycardia
3. constipation
4. heat intolerance
5. mild tremors
6. nervousness

a. 1, 4, 5, 6
b. 2, 3, 5
c. 3, 6
d. 4, 5

94. During the first day after delivery, a nurse assesses a client's fundus and notices that it feels boggy. Which is the first action that the nurse should perform?

a. Document the "boggy" fundus.
b. Have the client void.
c. Massage the fundus.
d. Notify the physician.

95. A client is diagnosed with antisocial personality disorder. The nurse should assess the client for which of the following? Select all that apply.

1. anxiety
2. risk for harming self
3. risk for harming others
4. substance abuse

a. 1, 2, 3
b. 2, 3, 4
c. 1, 3, 4
d. 1, 2, 4

96. A nurse is assessing a client's Babinski reflex. On the illustration, which location indicates the point where the nurse should place the tongue blade to begin the stroke of the foot?

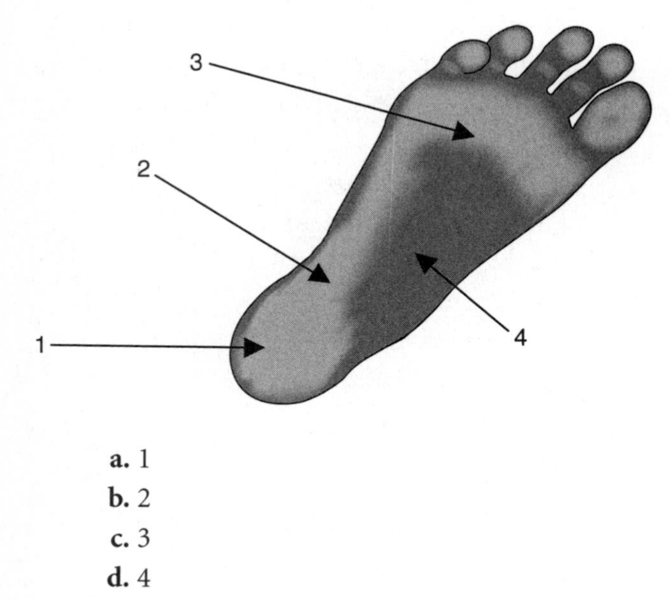

a. 1
b. 2
c. 3
d. 4

97. During a nurse's morning assessment of a client, the nurse notes that the client's abdominal girth has increased since the previous shift. The nurse also recognizes that the client has increased ascites. The client's vital signs are a temperature of 37.3°C, a heart rate of 118 bpm, shallow respirations of 26 breaths per minute, a blood pressure of 130/77 mm Hg, and an SpO_2 of 89% on room air. Given these assessment findings, which of the following actions should receive priority by the nurse?
a. Perform assessment of heart sounds.
b. Elevate the head of the bed.
c. Obtain an order for blood cultures.
d. Prepare for a paracentesis.

98. A nurse is caring for a client who is to receive eyedrops as well as eye ointment in the left eye. Which of the following demonstrates appropriate administration of these medications?
a. Administer the eyedrops first, followed by the eye ointment.
b. Administer the eyedrops, wait 10 minutes, and then administer the eye ointment.
c. Administer the eye ointment first, followed by the eyedrops.
d. Administer the eye ointment, wait 10 minutes, and then administer the eyedrops.

99. A primigravida comes to the office for a routine prenatal visit. The nurse assesses the fetal heart rate as 130 beats per minute. The nurse should
a. anticipate that the woman will need an ultrasound.
b. document the fetal heart rate as 130 beats per minute.
c. reassess the fetal heart rate.
d. turn the mother on her left side.

100. A physician orders a Guthrie test for an infant. The child's mother asks the nurse about the test. The nurse should answer that it is a screening test for
a. cystic fibrosis.
b. Down syndrome.
c. phenylketonuria.
d. spina bifida.

101. A client is being cared for in a burn unit after suffering partial-thickness burns. The client's laboratory work reveals a positive wound culture for gram-negative bacteria. The physician orders silver sulfadiazine (Silvadene) to be applied to the client's burns. The nurse provides information to the client about the medication. Which of the following statements made by the client indicates a lack of understanding about this treatment?

a. "This medication is an antibacterial."
b. "This medication will be applied directly to the wounds."
c. "This medication will stain my skin permanently."
d. "This medication will help my burns heal."

102. A client is being released from the same-day surgery center following glaucoma surgery. Which of the following is correct for the nurse to include in the discharge instructions related to home care?

a. Add extra lighting in the home.
b. Decrease daily fluid intake.
c. Decrease the amount of active exercise.
d. Wear dark sunglasses in the sunlight.

103. A nurse is performing the admission assessment on a client diagnosed with schizophrenia. Upon assessment, the client imitates the nurse's movements. The nurse should document this as

a. aphasia.
b. ataxia.
c. echolalia.
d. echopraxia.

104. A primigravida is in the active phase of labor. When the nurse performs Leopold's maneuver, the fetal head is palpated at position 4, as illustrated. The nurse then concludes that the fetus is in which of the following positions?

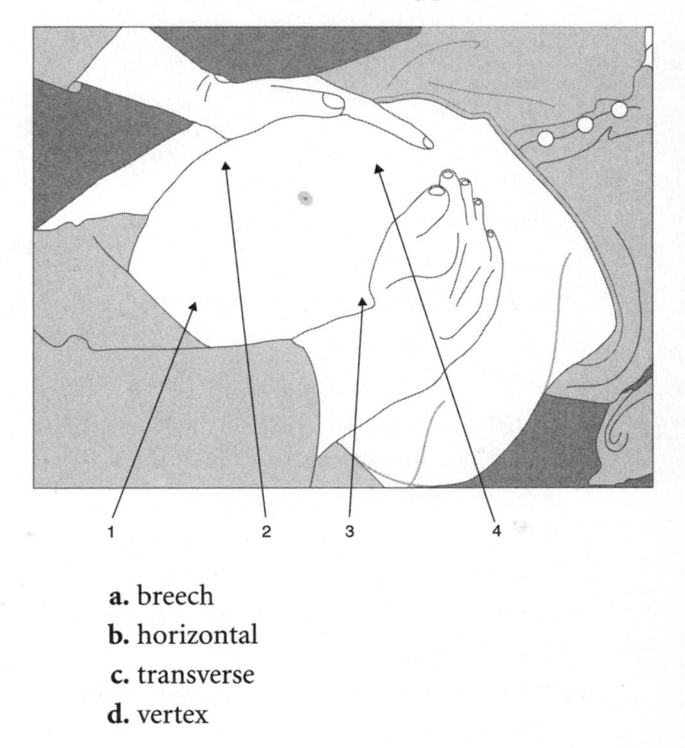

a. breech
b. horizontal
c. transverse
d. vertex

105. A nurse is caring for a 40-year-old male client diagnosed with essential hypertension. To diagnose essential hypertension, the nurse understands that the client's blood pressure readings were consistently at or above which of the following?

a. 125/90 mm Hg
b. 132/85 mm Hg
c. 140/90 mm Hg
d. 168/80 mm Hg

106. A nurse is caring for a client with a right-arm arteriovenous fistula. The nurse recognizes that the client is at risk for developing arterial steal syndrome. The nurse assesses the client for which of the following manifestations that will confirm the diagnosis of this syndrome?
a. aching pain, pallor, and edema of the right arm
b. edema and reddish discoloration of the right arm
c. pain in the right arm, arm pallor, and diminished pulse
d. warmth, pain in the right hand, and redness

107. A nurse is caring for a client who has a newly performed colostomy. After participating in colostomy-care sessions with the nurse and receiving support from his spouse, the client has decided to change the colostomy pouch alone. Which of the following behaviors indicates that the client is beginning to accept the change in body image?
a. The client rarely speaks about the recent surgery.
b. The client requests that his spouse leave the room.
c. The client tightly closes his eyes when the abdomen is exposed.
d. The client touches the affected body part.

108. The father of a toddler admitted for a colostomy due to Hirschsprung's disease is afraid that he will not be able to manage the ostomy. An appropriate response by the nurse is
a. "The home care nurse will help."
b. "Everyone is a little afraid at first."
c. "You can do it. I have watched you do it."
d. "You are worried about managing the ostomy."

109. The nurse correctly identifies the following rhythm strip as which of the following?

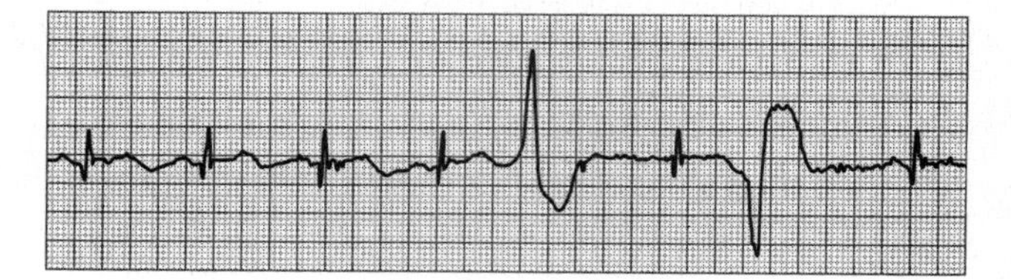

a. sinus rhythm with premature atrial contractions (PACs)
b. sinus rhythm with second-degree atrioventricular (AV) block—Mobitz I
c. sinus rhythm with premature ventricular contractions (PVCs)
d. ventricular pacing

110. A pregnant client who is five weeks gestation comes to the emergency room with a suspected ectopic pregnancy. Based on this, what would the nurse expect to find upon assessment?
a. cervical dilation
b. hemorrhage
c. nausea and vomiting
d. unilateral pelvic pain

111. A laboring client asks for pain medication and an order is written for Stadol. Prior to administering the medication, the nurse should assess the client's
a. fundal height.
b. heart rate.
c. lochia.
d. respirations.

112. A nurse is caring for a client on the oncology unit. The client states, "I am so itchy." The nurse relays to the client that the pruritus is probably caused by the cancer or the treatments. Which of the following nursing interventions is most appropriate for the nurse to implement?
a. administration of antihistamines
b. administration of topical steroids
c. dressing the bed with silk sheets
d. medicated baths *pro re nata* (PRN)

113. A client is admitted to a psychiatric hospital with a conversion disorder. The client is experiencing an inability to move his right arm. However, the client does not seem to be appropriately concerned about this, nor does the client display any symptoms of anxiety. The nurse knows that the client is exhibiting
a. catatonic excitement.
b. catonic stupor.
c. la belle indifference.
d. pseudoneurologic manifestation.

114. A client presents to the community health center 48 hours after receiving a Mantoux skin test for evaluation with a positive response to the test. The nurse understands that the finding indicates that the client
a. is actively immune to tuberculosis.
b. has produced an immune response.
c. has an active case of tuberculosis.
d. will develop full-blown tuberculosis.

115. A client has just completed delivering a stillborn infant. What intervention should the nurse complete first?
a. Provide the mother with an opportunity to hold the infant.
b. Put a discrete sign or symbol on the door alerting healthcare personnel of the fetal death.
c. Remove the infant from the room.
d. Refer the mother to a support group.

116. A nurse is planning care for a client who is exhibiting pain in the left lower extremity eight weeks after fracturing the tibia, even though the fracture is completely healed and all other complications have been ruled out. The client rates the pain at a level 6 on a 10-point scale. The nurse's plan of care should include interventions for a client with
a. hypochondria.
b. pain disorder.
c. conversion disorder.
d. body dysmorphic disorder.

117. A nurse is supervising a graduate nurse during the insertion of a urinary catheter in a female client diagnosed with fluid overload. The graduate nurse should advance the catheter how far into the urethra?
a. $\frac{1}{2}$″ (1 cm)
b. 2″ (5 cm)
c. 3.6″ (15 cm)
d. 3.8″ (20 cm)

118. A nurse is caring for a client complaining of abdominal pain. While assessing the client's abdomen, where should the nurse place his hand to palpate the liver?

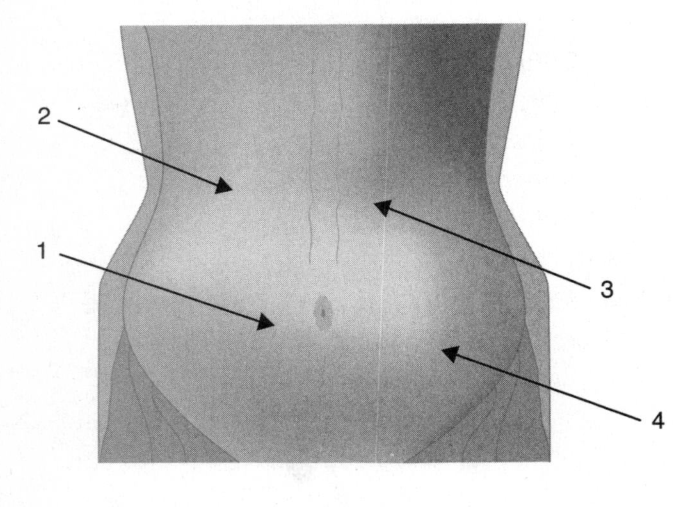

a. 1
b. 2
c. 3
d. 4

119. A nurse is providing education to a caregiver on management of a child's pinworms. The nurse should include instructions for which of the following?
a. administration of tinidazole (Tindamax)
b. monitoring for abdominal cramping
c. prevention of dehydration
d. proper hand washing technique

120. A nurse just received the morning laboratory results for a client with chronic renal failure. The client's serum calcium level is 8.4 mg/dL, and the client's serum phosphorus level is 4.0 mg/dL. Given these laboratory results, the nurse should monitor the client for the development of which the following? Select all that apply.
1. cardiac arrhythmias
2. constipation
3. decreased clotting times
4. drowsiness and lethargy
5. fractures
6. Trousseau sign

a. 3, 4
b. 2, 3, 5
c. 4, 5, 6
d. 1, 4, 5, 6

121. A client who is breast-feeding her infant was discharged from the hospital two days ago after a healthy vaginal delivery. The client calls the clinic nurse and states that her right breast is swollen, painful, and warm to the touch, and that she has a temperature of 101°F. The nurse should instruct the client to
a. discontinue breast-feeding and use warm compresses on the breast.
b. go to the emergency room.
c. make a clinic appointment for next week.
d. make a clinic appointment for today.

122. A nurse is caring for a female client who is diagnosed with a sexual pain disorder. The nurse should assess for which of the following? Select all that apply.

1. aversion
2. dyspareunia
3. hypoactive desire
4. vaginisimus

a. 1, 4
b. 2, 3
c. 2, 4
d. 3, 4

123. A client is in for her first prenatal visit. She asks the nurse when she will be able to hear her baby's heartbeat. The nurse knows that the fetal heart rate can be detected by

a. Doppler in the second month.
b. Doppler in the third month.
c. stethoscope in the third month.
d. stethoscope in the fourth month.

124. A nurse is assessing the level of consciousness of a client who has suffered a head injury. The client's Glasgow Coma Scale score is 15. Which of the following responses did the nurse assess in this client to arrive at a score of 15? Select all that apply.

1. bradycardia and hypotension
2. incomprehensible sounds
3. motor response to localized pain
4. orientation to person, place, and time
5. spontaneous eye opening
6. unequal pupil size

a. 1, 2
b. 4, 5
c. 1, 3, 6
d. 2, 3, 5

125. A child comes to the emergency room after drinking turpentine. Assessment findings include burning sensation in the throat and drooling. The priority intervention for the nurse is to

a. administer activated charcoal.
b. administer a cathartic.
c. dilute the corrosive with milk.
d. induce vomiting.

126. A graduate nurse is reviewing ECG rhythm tracings with her preceptor. The graduate nurse would correctly identify the following rhythm as

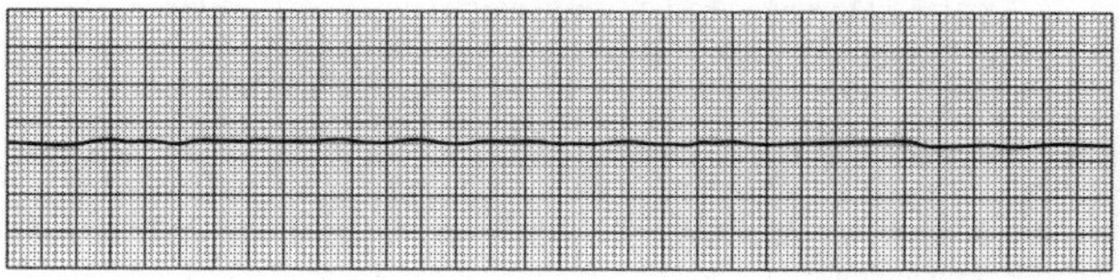

a. artifact.
b. asystole.
c. coarse ventricular fibrillation.
d. fine ventricular fibrillation.

127. A client is being treated in the ICU after experiencing premature ventricular contractions. The nurse has initiated an IV infusion of lidocaine hydrochloride. Upon assessment, the client is experiencing periods of excitation. Which of the following is also considered a side effect of IV lidocaine administration?

a. lethargy
b. palpitations
c. tinnitus
d. urinary frequency

128. A nurse is caring for a client at 38 weeks gestation who has been diagnosed with eclampsia. The client begins to complain of upper right quadrant abdominal pain and begins to vomit. The client's blood work reveals that the liver enzymes are elevated. Which action should NOT be performed by the nurse at this time?

a. administration of magnesium sulfate per order
b. fetal monitoring
c. palpation of the client's abdomen
d. preparation of the client for delivery

129. A client is being treated in the emergency department for an ischemic stroke. The client is ordered to receive a tissue plasminogen activator (t-PA). In preparation to give this medication, the nurse should complete which of the following first?

a. Ask what medications the client is taking at present.
b. Complete a history and physical assessment.
c. Determine the onset time of the stroke.
d. Identify if the client is scheduled for surgery.

130. A nurse is providing nutritional education for an alcoholic client. The nurse knows that alcohol inhibits the absorption of thiamine. Which of the following foods is a good source of thiamine?

a. apples
b. fish
c. green beans
d. nuts

131. A nurse is caring for a client whose status is post–total laryngectomy. The nurse should include which of the following in the client's plan of care?

a. Ensure the tracheostomy cuff is fully inflated.
b. Develop an alternative form of communication.
c. Encourage oral feedings as soon as possible.
d. Keep the client flat in bed.

132. A child is admitted to the pediatric unit with decreased white blood cells. The father asks the nurse if she thinks that the child has leukemia. An appropriate response by the nurse is

a. "I am not sure."
b. "The test results are not back yet."
c. "Are you concerned that your child has leukemia?"
d. "Ask your doctor when he comes in."

133. A nurse has just assessed a client's blood pressure one day postdelivery. After obtaining a reading of 120/72 mm Hg, the nurse removes the blood pressure cuff and notices that the client's arm is ecchymotic in the area where the blood pressure cuff was located. The nurse should

a. monitor the client's intake and output.
b. notify the physician.
c. place the cuff on the client more loosely next time.
d. retake the blood pressure on the other arm.

134. A client is admitted to a nursing unit with a diagnosis of pneumonia. Upon assessment, the client has a productive cough and is diaphoretic with a temperature of 103.2°F. Which of the following actions should the nurse include in the care for this client?

a. frequent linen changes
b. providing a bedpan for the client frequently
c. nasotracheal suctioning
d. repositioning the client every four hours

135. A nurse is assessing a client who overdosed on cocaine. The nurse assesses for which of the following? Select all that apply.

1. cardiac arrhythmias
2. increased blood pressure
3. diarrhea
4. pupil constriction

a. 1, 2, 3
b. 1, 2, 4
c. 2, 3, 4
d. 1, 3, 4

136. A client being cared for on a medical-surgical unit has had a colectomy nine hours ago. The client has just used a patient-controlled analgesia (PCA) pump to administer morphine for pain. Additionally, the client has been repositioned for comfort and has stable vital signs. What should the nurse do next?

a. Apply 2L oxygen via nasal cannula.
b. Dim the room lights.
c. Check on the client's family.
d. Reassess the client's vital signs.

137. A nurse receives the laboratory results for a client who is receiving IV antineoplastic medications. Which of the following serum laboratory results would necessitate that the nurse implement bleeding precautions?

a. ammonia level: 30 mcg/dL
b. clotting time: 15 minutes
c. platelet count: 50,000/mm^3
d. white blood cell count: 7,000/mm^3

138. A nurse is providing discharge instructions for a client who is receiving sulfisoxazole. Which of the following should be included in the instructions?

a. Decrease the dose of medication when symptoms are improving.
b. Maintain a high fluid intake.
c. Notify the physician immediately if urine turns dark brown.
d. Restrict fluid intake.

139. A nurse is planning a health-education seminar to teenagers on acne. The nurse's teaching should include which of the following? Select all that apply.

1. avoidance of popping an acne pimple
2. application of topical creams
3. sebum production decreases in teen years
4. use of birth control with Accutane

a. 1, 2, 3
b. 1, 3, 4
c. 1, 2, 4
d. 2, 3, 4

140. A nurse is caring for a client with myasthenia gravis. The client has become increasingly weaker since the nurse's earlier assessment. The physician prepares to identify whether the client is reacting to an overdose of medication (cholinergic crisis) or an increasing severity of the disease (myasthenic crisis). An injection of edrophonium (Tensilon) is administered. Which of the following would indicate the client is in cholinergic crisis?

a. complaints of muscle spasms
b. improvement of the client's weakness
c. no change in the client's condition
d. temporary worsening of the condition

141. A nurse is caring for a client with a history of diabetes and vascular dementia. To assist in the prevention of further cognitive changes, the nurse's plan of care should include which of the following? Select all that apply.

1. administration of Aricept
2. a diet high in thiamine
3. increased exercise
4. monitoring client's glucose

a. 1, 2
b. 2, 3
c. 3, 4
d. 1, 4

142. A nurse is reviewing histamine (H_2)-receptor antagonist medications with a graduate nurse. The graduate nurse correctly identifies which of the following medications as H_2-receptor antagonists? Select all that apply.

1. cimetidine (Tagamet)
2. famotidine (Pepcid)
3. lansoprazole (Prevacid)
4. nizatidine (Axid)
5. ranitidine (Zantac)

a. 1, 5
b. 2, 4
c. 1, 2, 4, 5
d. 2, 3, 4, 5

143. A nursing manager is conducting rounds on the labor and delivery unit. Currently, there are four clients in labor. One client is at station 0, the second client is at station −1, the third client is at station +3, and the fourth client is at station −3. Based only on this information, the manager anticipates which client to deliver first?

a. client at station 0
b. client at station −1
c. client at station +3
d. client at station −3

144. A nurse is caring for a client who is ordered for a magnetic resonance imaging (MRI). The nurse should advise the client that which of the following actions would pose a threat to the client during the MRI?

a. the client asking questions during the scan
b. the client lying still during the scan
c. the client hearing a thumping sound during the scan
d. the client wearing a ring and bracelet during the scan

145. A child with a history of hydrocephalus is admitted to the pediatric unit for a shunt replacement. Postoperatively, the child becomes irritable and combative, and complains of a headache. The nurse's first intervention is to

a. document the findings.
b. administer Tylenol.
c. notify the physician.
d. utilize restraints.

146. A nurse for the evening shift has just received report on her clients. After making initial rounds, which of the following clients will the nurse plan to care for first?
a. a client requiring colostomy irrigation
b. a client requiring a chest X-ray
c. a client with a fever who is diaphoretic
d. a client who just received pain medication

147. A charge nurse is preparing nursing assignments for the daylight shift. Which of the following clients are appropriate for the nurse to assign to a licensed practical nurse (LPN) to provide client care? Select all that apply.
1. a client receiving total parenteral nutrition (TPN)
2. a client who had an appendectomy two days ago
3. a client with diverticulitis who requires teaching about medications
4. a client who is experiencing an exacerbation of ulcerative colitis
5. a client with an intestinal obstruction who needs a nasogastric (NG) tube inserted

a. 1, 5
b. 2, 4
c. 1, 2, 5
d. 2, 3, 4

148. A nurse is caring for a client with multiple past admissions to the hospital for hypoglycemia. Which of the following instructions should the nurse reinforce with the client to help decrease the episodes of hypoglycemia?
a. Consume a candy bar when lightheadedness occurs.
b. Eat a high-protein, low-carbohydrate diet, and avoid fasting.
c. Increase foods high in saturated fats and fast in the afternoon.
d. Take iron supplements while increasing foods high in vitamins B and D.

149. A nurse is preparing to administer eardrops to a child who is three years old. The nurse should administer the eardrops by gently pulling the pinna
a. down and back.
b. down and outward.
c. up and back.
d. up and outward.

150. A nurse is caring for a toddler with a history of bronchopulmonary dysplasia who was admitted due to respiratory infection. The nurse should anticipate physician orders for all of the following EXCEPT
a. antibiotics.
b. steroids.
c. bronchodilators.
d. a surfactant.

151. A nurse is preparing to document a child's weight in kilograms. The child weighs 62 pounds. The nurse should document the child's weight as
a. 26.96 kg
b. 28.18 kg
c. 136.40 kg
d. 138 kg

152. A nurse is assigned to care for a client whose cultural background is different from her own. To address the situation, the nurse should do which of the following? Select all that apply.
1. Ask the client if there are cultural or religious requirements that should be considered in the plan of care.
2. Explain the nurse's beliefs so that the client will understand the differences.
3. Recognize that all cultures experience pain in the same way.
4. Respect the client's cultural beliefs.
5. Understand that nonverbal cues, such as eye contact, may have a different meaning in different cultures.

a. 1, 5
b. 1, 4, 5
c. 2, 3, 4
d. 1, 2, 3, 4, 5

153. A nurse is caring for a client with depersonalization disorder. Which of the following would the nurse expect to find?
a. hallucinations
b. feeling detached from the body
c. loss of memories
d. anxiety

154. A client diagnosed with lung cancer has received external beam radiation therapy. The nurse caring for the client should assess for which of the following?
a. diarrhea
b. dysphasia
c. improved energy level
d. normal white blood cell count

155. A client is admitted to the medical-surgical unit with a diagnosis of Addison's disease. The nurse assigned to this client's care should review laboratory reports for which of the following conditions?
a. decreased BUN level
b. hypernatremia
c. hypoglycemia
d. hypocalcemia

156. During a home visit to a Hispanic client and her infant one week after delivery, the nurse notices dark blue marks on the neonate's buttocks. The nurse should
a. document these as Mongolian spots.
b. document these as Montgomery spots.
c. notify the physician.
d. suspect abuse.

157. A client in the active phase of labor is at 38 weeks gestation and has a history of preeclampsia. As she is ambulating to the bathroom, the client experiences severe abdominal pain and a gush of dark red vaginal bleeding. The nurse should implement appropriate nursing interventions for
a. placental abruption.
b. eclampsia.
c. HELLP syndrome.
d. placenta previa.

158. A nurse is caring for a client with delirium. Which of the following should the nurse's plan of care include? Select all that apply.
1. chemical restraint
2. cognition assessment
3. environmental stimulation
4. relaxation techniques

a. 1, 2
b. 2, 3
c. 3, 4
d. 2, 4

159. A child with cerebral palsy is documented to have diplegia. The nurse prepares to care for a child whose dysfunction is
a. equal in all four extremities.
b. greater in the lower extremities.
c. greater in the upper extremities.
d. involves one side of the body.

160. A nurse is assigned to a client with a 12-hour-old male infant. During report, the nurse was told that the client is in the taking-hold phase of Rubin's bonding phases. The nurse knows that during this phase it is appropriate to perform which intervention?
a. Assess for symptoms of depression in the mother.
b. Contact the physician to perform a circumcision on the infant.
c. Encourage the mother to verbalize her birthing experience.
d. Teach the mother basic infant care.

161. A client diagnosed with acute pancreatitis is being treated on a medical-surgical unit. Which of the following complications should the nurse look for in this client?
a. cirrhosis
b. duodenal ulcer
c. heart failure
d. pneumonia

162. A client has been recently diagnosed with Raynaud's phenomenon. To prevent recurrent vasospastic episodes, the nurse should instruct the client to complete which the following?
a. Elevate the hands and feet as much as possible.
b. Increase coffee intake to three cups per day.
c. Utilize a vibrating massage device on the hands.
d. Wear gloves while obtaining food from the freezer.

163. A nurse is caring for a client who had an abdominal perineal resection three days ago. Upon assessment, the nurse notes that the wound edges are not approximated and half of the incision has separated. The nurse should immediately take which of the following actions?
a. Apply an abdominal binder.
b. Apply a strip of tape to the incision.
c. Cover the wound with a moist sterile dressing.
d. Irrigate the wound with sterile water.

164. Growth and development principles set forth that growth occurs in a proximodistal direction. The nurse knows this means that a child will gain control of
a. arm then finger movement.
b. arm then leg movement.
c. finger then arm movement.
d. leg then arm movement.

165. A nurse is working with a three-year-old child. The child states that his stuffed animal told him to put his toys away. The nurse knows that this is a normal occurrence in which of Piaget's stages of development?
a. concrete operational thought
b. formal operational thought
c. preoperational thought
d. sensorimotor period

Answers

1. b. The nurse should relay to the client that dizziness (2), headache (3), and hypotension (5) are all common adverse effects of lisinopril and other ACE inhibitors. Choices **a** and **c** are incorrect. Lisinopril may cause diarrhea, not constipation (1). Lisinopril does not cause hyperglycemia (4) or impotence (6). Choice **d** is incorrect. Lisinopril does not cause hyperglycemia (4) or impotence (6).
Category: Physiological Integrity: Pharmacological and Parenteral Therapies
Subcategory: Adult: Cardiovascular Disorders

2. a. During true labor, the cervix dilates and effaces. Choice **b** is incorrect. True labor contractions will continue to increase in strength and frequency when sitting. Choice **c** is incorrect. Braxton-Hicks contractions, not true labor contractions, will decrease with ambulation. Choice **d** is incorrect. Lightening refers to the dropping of the fetus into the pelvic cavity. It is not a sign of true labor.
Category: Health Promotion and Maintenance
Subcategory: Maternal Infant: Intrapartum

3. c. Area 3 is considered the QRS complex. Choice **a** is incorrect. Area 1 is considered the ST segment. Choice **b** is incorrect. Area 2 is considered the PR interval. Choice **d** is incorrect. Area 4 is considered the ST interval.
Category: Physiological Integrity: Physiological Adaptation
Subcategory: Adult: Cardiovascular Disorders

4. a. The deltoid is an appropriate site to administer an IM injection to a toddler. Choice **b** is incorrect. This site is appropriate to administer a subcutaneous injection but not an IM injection. Choice **c** is incorrect. The dorsogluteal site is an appropriate site to administer an IM injection for children preschool age and older but not for toddlers. Choice **d** is incorrect. The ventrogluteal site is an appropriate site to administer an IM injection for children preschool age and older but not for toddlers.
Category: Physiological Integrity: Pharmacological and Parenteral Therapies
Subcategory: Pediatrics: Medication Administration

5. a. The nurse should instruct the client to chew his or her food thoroughly. This will aid in digestion as well as prevent obstruction. Choice **b** is incorrect. It is unnecessary for the nurse to instruct the client to eat six small meals a day. Choice **c** is incorrect. It is unnecessary for the client to restrict fluid intake. The client should remain adequately hydrated. Choice **d** is incorrect. The client is usually placed on a regular diet, but is encouraged to use caution about eating high-fiber, high-cellulose foods (e.g., nuts, popcorn, corn, peas, tomatoes), as these foods may swell in the intestine and cause an obstruction.
Category: Physiological Integrity: Basic Care and Comfort
Subcategory: Adult: Gastrointestinal Disorders

6. d. Terminally ill clients often describe feelings of isolation because they feel ignored. The terminally ill client may also sense any discomfort that family and friends feel in the client's presence. Appropriate nursing interventions include spending time with the client, encouraging discussion about feelings, and answering questions openly and honestly. Choices **a**, **b**, and **c** are incorrect. Reducing the client's fears is secondary to lessening the client's feelings of isolation.
Category: Psychosocial Integrity
Subcategory: Adult: Oncology Disorders

7. c. Remeron is used to treat clients with depression. Choice **a** is incorrect. Medications for anxiety disorders include benzodiazepines, barbiturates, and sedatives. Choice **b** is incorrect. Medications for bipolar disorder include lithium. Choice **d** is incorrect. Medications for sleep disorders include barbiturates and sedatives.
Category: Physiological Integrity: Pharmacological and Parenteral Therapies
Subcategory: Mental Health: Medications

8. b. The client should void prior to initiating the therapy so that she is able to maintain a supine position for up to two hours after the medication is administered. Choice **a** is incorrect. Prostaglandin E is administered vaginally, not intravenously. Choice **c** is incorrect. Stomach cramping is an adverse reaction to the medication and therefore would not occur until the medication is administered. Choice **d** is incorrect. The client should be positioned in a supine position after the medication is administered.
Category: Physiological Integrity: Pharmacological and Parenteral Therapies
Subcategory: Maternal Infant: Maternal Medications

9. b. Pain is common during the first few exchanges because of peritoneal irritation; however, the pain usually disappears after one to two weeks of regular treatments. Choice **a** incorrect. The amount of solution being infused should not be decreased. It should be explained to client that the pain will decrease after more exchanges. Choice **c** is incorrect. The infusion rate or infusion amounts should not be slowed down; pain during the first one to two sessions is common. Choice **d** is incorrect. The dialysis session should not be immediately discontinued. It should be explained to client that the pain will decrease after more exchanges.
Category: Physiological Integrity: Physiological Adaptation
Subcategory: Adult: Renal Disorders

10. a. To perform Barlow's maneuver, the nurse places the index and middle fingers on the greater trochanters and the thumbs at the inner thigh inguinal creases. The hip is then gently adducted, or moved inward. Choice **b** is incorrect. Chadwick's sign refers to a bluish discoloration of the vagina, cervix, and labia during pregnancy. Choice **c** is incorrect. Hegar's sign refers to a softening of the cervix during pregnancy. Choice **d** is incorrect. While Ortolani's maneuver is also used to assess for hip dysplasia, the nurse performs the maneuver by abducting the newborn's hips, not adducting, which is performed in Barlow's maneuver.
Category: Health Promotion and Maintenance
Subcategory: Pediatrics: Musculoskeletal Disorders

11. **c.** Beractant is a lung surfactant administered to infants to prevent or treat respiratory distress syndrome in preterm infants. Choice **a** is incorrect. Asthma is treated with bronchodilators or steroids. Beractant is a lung surfactant. Choice **b** is incorrect. Neonatal croup is treated with bronchodilators and steroids. Beractant is a lung surfactant. Choice **d** is incorrect. While there are ways to reduce the risk for Sudden Infant Death Syndrome, there is no medication available at this time to prevent it.
Category: Physiological Integrity: Pharmacological and Parenteral Therapies
Subcategory: Maternal Infant: Neonatal Complications

12. **a.** Tamoxifen can increase calcium, cholesterol, and triglyceride levels. Prior to the administration of this drug, the nurse should obtain a complete blood count and platelet count. Serum calcium levels should also be assessed and monitored periodically during the therapy. The nurse should assess for signs and symptoms of hypercalcemia, which include increased urine volume, excessive thirst, constipation, vomiting, nausea, hypotonicity of muscles, flank pain, and deep bone pain. Choice **b** is incorrect. The glucose level does not need to be monitored in relation to the administration of this medication. Choice **c** is incorrect. The potassium level does not need to be monitored related to the administration of this medication. Choice **d** is incorrect. The prothrombin time does not need to be monitored in relation to the administration of this medication.
Category: Physiological Integrity: Pharmacological and Parenteral Therapies
Subcategory: Adult: Oncology Disorders

13. **b.** Lying on the left side allows the enema solution to flow downward by gravity into the rectum and sigmoid colon. Choices **a**, **c**, and **d** are incorrect. These are not appropriate positions for self-administration of an enema.
Category: Safe and Effective Care Environment: Safety and Infection Control
Subcategory: Adult: Oncology Disorders

14. **c.** The expected assessment findings would include confusion (2) and somnolence (4). Choice **a** is incorrect. The expected assessment findings would include somnolence (4) but not hyperactivity (1). Choice **b** is incorrect. The expected assessment findings would include confusion (2) and decreased, not increased, reflexes (3). Choice **d** is incorrect. The client with benzodiazepine toxicity would not exhibit hyperactivity (1) or increased reflexes (3).
Category: Physiological Integrity: Pharmacological and Parenteral Therapies
Subcategory: Mental Health: Medications

15. **b.** The client is in false labor and should return home. Choice **a** is incorrect. The client is in false labor; therefore, instructing the client to ambulate in the halls is inappropriate. Choice **c** is incorrect. The client is in false labor and should not be admitted at this time. Choice **d** is incorrect. The client is in false labor; therefore, preparing for a cesarean section is not appropriate.
Category: Health Promotion and Maintenance
Subcategory: Maternal Infant: Intrapartum

16. **d.** In addition to not lifting heavy objects (2), the client should also be instructed to avoid lifting the arm on the operative side above shoulder level for one week postinsertion; prolonged immobilization is not required. Upon discharge, it is important for the nurse to teach the client how to take and record his or her pulse daily (5). Choices **a**, **b**, and **c** are incorrect. The pacemaker metal casing does not set off airport security alarms, so there is no need to avoid air travel (1). Microwave ovens are safe to use and do not alter pacemaker function (3). It generally takes up to two months for the incision site to heal and for the patient to regain full range of motion, but prolonged immobilization (4) is not required.
Category: Physiological Integrity: Reduction of Risk Potential
Subcategory: Adult: Cardiovascular Disorders

17. **b.** An overriding aorta (2), pulmonary stenosis (4), right ventricular hypertrophy (5), and ventral septal defect (6) are the four defects associated with tetralogy of Fallot. Choices **a** and **d** are incorrect. Left ventricular hypertrophy (1) occurs with congestive heart failure, and patent ductus arteriosus (3) occurs when the ductus arteriosus fails to close after birth. Choice **c** is incorrect. Patent ductus arteriosus (3) occurs when the ductus arteriosus fails to close after birth.
Category: Physiological Integrity: Physiological Adaptation
Subcategory: Pediatrics: Cardiovascular Disorders

18. **c.** The gross motor ability to pull up into a standing position usually develops around 10 to 12 months of age. Choice **a** is incorrect. The fine motor skill to transfer objects from hand to hand develops around four to six months of age. Choice **b** is incorrect. The cognitive skill to play peekaboo usually develops around 10 to 12 months of age. Choice **d** is incorrect. The social/adaptive skill to use a fork usually develops around 18 to 24 months of age.
Category: Safe and Effective Care Environment: Management of Care
Subcategory: Pediatrics: Growth and Development

19. **c.** Providing the client with a piece of hard candy will aid in eliminating thirst and maintain the fluid restriction. Choice **a** is incorrect. Reinforcing the need for maintaining the fluid restriction does not address the client's needs. Choice **b** is incorrect. It is nontherapeutic to ignore the client's request for fluids. Choice **d** is incorrect. The nurse is aware that the client must adhere to the ordered fluid restriction and that the physician will not alter the order. It would be inappropriate for the nurse to provide the client with more fluids than prescribed. This may result in fluid overload, which could lead to an emergency hemodialysis session.
Category: Physiological Integrity: Basic Care and Comfort
Subcategory: Adult: Renal Disorders

20. a. Behavioral therapy uses learning principles to effect changes in behavior by focusing on the consequences of actions. Choice **b** is incorrect. Cognitive therapy focuses on replacing clients' negative or irrational beliefs. Choice **c** is incorrect. Crisis therapy focuses on identification of immediate coping patterns. Choice **d** is incorrect. Milieu therapy incorporates a planned use of the treatment environment as part of the therapy.
Category: Psychosocial Integrity
Subcategory: Mental Health: Therapy

21. a. Decerebrate posturing occurs in clients with damage to the upper brain stem, midbrain, or pons, and is demonstrated clinically by arching of the back, rigid extension of the extremities, pronation of the arms, and plantar flexion of the feet. Choices **b** and **d** are incorrect. These answers do not describe decerebrate posturing. Choice **c** is incorrect. This answer describes decorticate posturing.
Category: Physiological Integrity: Physiological Adaptation
Subcategory: Adult: Neurological Disorders

22. a. The child's weight is in the 5th percentile and his height in the 90th percentile. The child needs to increase his caloric intake, and an appropriate intervention for this is to increase nutritious snacking. Choice **b** is incorrect. The child's weight is in the 5th percentile and his height is in the 90th percentile. This does not indicate a need for increased physical activity. Choice **c** is incorrect. Decreased caloric intake would cause the child's weight to drop even further and cause further disproportion between the child's height and weight. Choice **d** is incorrect. The child's weight is in the 5th percentile while his height is in the 90th percentile. While setting limits on television viewing is important for all children, it would not help the child to increase his weight appropriately.
Category: Health Promotion and Maintenance
Subcategory: Pediatrics: Growth and Development

23. d. The client with a soft, boggy uterus is at risk for postpartum hemorrhage. The nurse should attend to this client first by gently massaging the client's fundus. Choice **a** is incorrect. The soreness is most likely related to incorrect latching on of the infant. The nurse can work with this client the next time she goes to feed the infant. Choice **b** is incorrect. A first-degree perineal laceration is usually small and does not involve the muscles. This type of tear usually heals quickly and causes little or minimal discomfort. Therefore, this client does not need immediate attention. Choice **c** is incorrect. Lochia rubra is the expected finding for the first two to three days in the postpartum period. This client does not need to be seen first by the nurse.
Category: Safe and Effective Care Environment: Management of Care
Subcategory: Maternal Infant: Maternal Complications: Postpartum

24. c. It indicates the location of Erb's point, where the aortic and pulmonic valve sounds radiate. Choice **a** is incorrect. It indicates the location of the aortic valve sounds. Choice **b** is incorrect. It indicates the location of the pulmonic valve sounds. Choice **d** is incorrect. It indicates the location of the mitral valve sounds.
Category: Health Promotion and Maintenance
Subcategory: Adult: Cardiovascular Disorders

25. d. The client may require blood products, depending on laboratory values and severity of bleeding; therefore, availability of blood product should be confirmed by calling the blood bank (3). The hemoglobin and hematocrit levels should be assessed to evaluate blood loss; an elevated INR and PTT and a decreased platelet count increase the risk for postoperative bleeding and must be evaluated (4). Close monitoring of blood loss from the mediastinal chest tube should also be completed (5). Choices **a**, **b**, and **c** are incorrect. Coumadin (1) is an anticoagulant that will increase bleeding and should be held postoperatively. It is necessary to obtain information on the type of valve replacement received. For a mechanical heart valve, the INR is kept at 2 to 3.5. Tissue valves do not require anticoagulation. Dopamine should not be initiated if the client is hypotensive from hypovolemia; a fluid volume assessment should always be completed first, and fluid resuscitation should be used prior to initiating an infusion of dopamine (2).
Category: Physiological Integrity: Physiological Adaptation
Subcategory: Adult: Cardiovascular Disorders

26. **d.** Clients receiving PN solutions are at risk for developing hypoglycemia. It is essential that the solution containing the highest amount of glucose should be hung until the new PN solution becomes available. Because PN solutions contain high glucose concentrations, the 10% dextrose in water is the best choice. Choices **a**, **b**, and **c** are incorrect. Clients receiving PN solutions are at risk for developing hypoglycemia. These solutions will not be as effective in decreasing the risk of hypoglycemia as 10% dextrose in water.
Category: Physiological Integrity: Pharmacological and Parenteral Therapies
Subcategory: Adult: Gastrointestinal Disorders

27. **d.** Resolution of emotional and self-esteem issues is the goal of group therapy. Choice **a** is incorrect. Assessment of family functioning is the goal of family therapy. Choice **b** is incorrect. Identification of immediate coping patterns is the goal of crisis intervention. Choice **c** is incorrect. Replacement of negative attitudes and behaviors is the goal of cognitive therapy.
Category: Psychosocial Integrity
Subcategory: Mental Health: Therapy

28. **c.** A patent ductus arteriosus is an abnormal opening between the aorta and pulmonary artery that causes blood from the aorta to be shunted to the pulmonary artery. Choice **a** is incorrect. This is a healthy tricuspid valve. Choice **b** is incorrect. This depicts a portion of the aorta that has developed normally. Choice **d** is incorrect. This is a normally formed mitral valve.
Category: Physiological Integrity: Physiological Adaptation
Subcategory: Pediatrics: Cardiovascular Disorders

29. **c.** Chadwick's sign, a bluish coloration of the vagina, cervix, and vulva is a probable sign of pregnancy. Choice **a** is incorrect. Breast tenderness is a presumptive sign of pregnancy. Choice **b** is incorrect. Missing a period is a presumptive sign of pregnancy. Choice **d** is incorrect. Fetal heart tones are a positive sign of pregnancy.
Category: Health Promotion and Maintenance
Subcategory: Maternal Infant: Antepartum

30. **c.** Miotic medications are used to lower the intraocular pressure, which then increases blood flow to the retina. This decreases retinal damage and loss of vision. Miotic medication also causes a contraction or constriction of the ciliary muscle and widens the trabecular meshwork. Choices **a**, **b**, and **d** are incorrect. These are not effects of miotic medications.
Category: Physiological Integrity: Pharmacological and Parenteral Therapies
Subcategory: Adult: Eye Disorders

31. **b.** Nursing priorities are generally classified as high, intermittent, and low. A pulse oximetry reading of 85% is well below the normal level (95% to 100%) and indicates the highest priority. Choice **a** is incorrect. The hemoglobin level is within the normal range (male: 14 to 18 gm/dL; female: 12 to 16 gm/dL), making this a low priority. Choice **c** is incorrect. The urine output is adequate, however marginal, which is an intermittent priority. Choice **d** is incorrect. The potassium level is within the normal range (3.5 to 5 mEq/L), which is a low priority.
Category: Safe and Effective Care Environment: Management of Care
Subcategory: Adult: Miscellaneous

32. d. The nurse should set defined times for the client to perform the compulsive action. This will assist the client in decreasing the amount of time spent engaged in the activity. Choice **a** is incorrect. Focusing the client's attention on the behavior will not help the client understand the underlying cause of the behavior or learn how to control the behavior. Choice **b** is incorrect. Ignoring the compulsive behavior will not help the client to understand the underlying cause of the behavior or learn how to control the behavior. Choice **c** is incorrect. Preventing the client from performing the compulsive action may cause an increase in the client's anxiety.
Category: Psychosocial Integrity
Subcategory: Mental Health: Therapy

33. c. If peritonitis is present, antibiotics may be added to the dialysate (1). Broad-spectrum antibiotics may be administered to prevent infection when a peritoneal catheter is inserted for peritoneal dialysis (2). Peritonitis, the most serious and common complication of peritoneal dialysis (4), is characterized by cloudy dialysate drainage, diffuse abdominal pain, and rebound tenderness (3). Choices **a** and **d** are incorrect. Utilizing septic technique, not simply clean technique (5), is an imperative measure to prevent peritonitis. Choice **b** is incorrect. It omits teachings 1 and 3.
Category: Safe and Effective Care Environment: Safety and Infection Control
Subcategory: Adult: Renal Disorders

34. b. Increased thirst and urination during pregnancy are symptoms of gestational diabetes. The nurse should assess for additional symptoms such as glycosuria. Choices **a**, **c**, and **d** are incorrect. These conditions are not symptoms of gestational diabetes.
Category: Physiological Integrity: Reduction of Risk Potential
Subcategory: Maternal Infant: Maternal Complications: Antepartum

35. b. Often, monthly prophylactic antibiotic therapy will be ordered for a child with rheumatic heart disease. Choice **a** is incorrect. Digoxin is to be given if the heart rate is greater than 60 bpm. Choice **c** is incorrect. Tylenol is not contraindicated for a child with rheumatic heart disease. Choice **d** is incorrect. Aspirin is not contraindicated for a child with rheumatic heart disease.
Category: Physiological Integrity: Physiological Adaptation
Subcategory: Pediatrics: Cardiovascular Disorders

36. c. It is necessary for clients on hemodialysis to monitor their fluid status between hemodialysis treatments or sessions. This is accomplished by recording intake and output and weight on a daily basis. The client on hemodialysis should not gain more than 1.1 pounds (0.5 kg) of weight per day. Choice **a** is incorrect. It is unnecessary for the client to record blood urea nitrogen and creatinine levels daily. The physician will order these laboratory tests as needed. Choice **b** is incorrect. It is unnecessary for the client to record daily living activities and periods of weakness. Choice **d** is incorrect. It is unnecessary for the client to record daily respiratory and heart rates.
Category: Health Promotion and Maintenance
Subcategory: Adult: Renal Disorders

37. b. Between 32 and 36 weeks gestation, visits are scheduled for every other week in a healthy pregnancy. Choice **a** is incorrect. Weekly prenatal visits are scheduled after week 36 in a healthy pregnancy. Choice **c** is incorrect. Prenatal visits are usually not scheduled every three weeks in a healthy pregnancy. Choice **d** is incorrect. Monthly prenatal visits are usually scheduled between 4 and 32 weeks gestation.
Category: Physiological Integrity: Reduction of Risk Potential
Subcategory: Maternal Infant: Antepartum

38. b. The cardiac telemetry strip is showing atrial fibrillation. Clients experiencing this rhythm are at risk for clot formation. The client will be discharged home on the oral anticoagulant Coumadin. Choice **a** is incorrect. Clients experiencing atrial fibrillation are at risk for clot formation. The client will be discharged home on the oral anticoagulant Coumadin, not aspirin. Choice **c** is incorrect. The client will be discharged home on the oral anticoagulant Coumadin, not heparin, which is administered intravenously. Choice **d** is incorrect. The client will be discharged home on the oral anticoagulant Coumadin, not Ticlid. Ticlopidine is used to reduce the risk of stroke in clients who have had a stroke or have had warning signs of a stroke and who cannot be treated with aspirin. Ticlopidine is also used along with aspirin to prevent blood clots from forming in coronary stents.
Category: Physiological Integrity: Pharmacological and Parenteral Therapies
Subcategory: Adult: Cardiovascular Disorders

39. b. The client is having difficulty with short-term memory, which is controlled by the temporal lobe. Choice **a** is incorrect. The client is having difficulty with short-term memory. The location indicated by this choice is the frontal lobe, which regulates decision making, problem solving, consciousness, and emotions. Choice **c** is incorrect. The client is having difficulty with short-term memory. The location indicated by this choice is the occipital lobe, which processes information related to vision. Choice **d** is incorrect. The client is having difficulty with short-term memory. The location indicated by this choice is the cerebellum, which controls movement and balance.
Category: Physiological Integrity: Physiological Adaptation
Subcategory: Mental Health: Cognitive Disorders

40. b. It would be normal for a five-year-old child to have abdominal breathing (1). Due to the thinness of the chest wall, it would also be normal for the child to have hyperresonant lung sounds (3). Choice **a** is incorrect. While it would be expected for the child to exhibit abdominal breathing (1), the anterior-to-posterior ratio would be expected to be 1:2, not 1:1 (2). Choice **c** is incorrect. Due to the thinness of a young child's chest wall, it is normal to have hyperresonant breath sounds (3). However, the expected anterior-to-posterior ratio in a five-year-old child would be 1:2, not 1:1 (2). Choice **d** is incorrect. The expected anterior-to-posterior ratio in a five-year-old child is 1:2, not 1:1 (2). The expected respiratory rate in a healthy five-year-old is 20 to 28 breaths per minute, not 14 breaths per minute (4).
Category: Physiological Integrity: Basic Care and Comfort
Subcategory: Pediatrics: Cardiovascular Disorders

41. c. An expected medical outcome in the treatment of a client diagnosed with ulcerative colitis is that the client maintains an ideal body weight. Choice **a** is incorrect. It is not assumed that a client with the diagnosis of ulcerative colitis will need an ileostomy. The decision to perform surgery depends on the extent of the disease and the severity of the client's symptoms. Choice **b** is incorrect. The client diagnosed with ulcerative colitis will experience episodes of diarrhea, not constipation. Choice **d** is incorrect. The client should maintain adequate hydration; thus hydration should be encouraged.
Category: Physiological Integrity: Basic Care and Comfort
Subcategory: Adult: Gastrointestinal Disorders

42. b. Diabetic neuropathy, cataracts, and glaucoma are common complications in diabetes, thus necessitating the nurse to complete an eye assessment and examination. The client's feet should also be examined at each client encounter, as the nurse will monitor for thickening, fissures, ulcers, and thickened nails. Choices **a**, **c**, and **d** are incorrect. Although the nurse should assess these parts of the body in a thorough examination, they are not pertinent to common diabetic complications.
Category: Physiological Integrity: Reduction of Risk Potential
Subcategory: Adult: Endocrine Disorders

43. b. It is important for clients diagnosed with gastrointestinal reflux to eat smaller, more frequent meals to help prevent recurrence. Choice **a** is incorrect. The client should not lie down until two to three hours after food consumption to prevent reflux from recurring. Choice **c** is incorrect. Fluid should be restricted with meals to decrease gastric distention and prevent reflux from recurring. Choice **d** is incorrect. The client should elevate the head of the bed approximately four to six inches when sleeping. This facilitates esophageal emptying and decreases episodes of reflux.
Category: Physiological Integrity: Reduction of Risk Potential
Subcategory: Adult: Gastrointestinal Disorders

44. **c.** The nurse should give the client one command at a time. Choices **a** and **b** are incorrect. The client will not be able to follow a two-step command. Choice **d** is incorrect. Although the nurse is giving the client one command at a time, the client is not being instructed to get dressed.
Category: Safe and Effective Care Environment: Management of Care
Subcategory: Mental Health: Cognitive Disorders

45. **a.** Pregnant women should avoid undercooked eggs and meats due to risk of salmonella infection. Choice **b** is incorrect. Healthy pregnant women do not need to limit their sodium intake. Choice **c** is incorrect. Pregnant women should limit their caffeine intake to 300 mg per day. Choice **d** is incorrect. Breads and cereals fortified with folic acid should be consumed by pregnant women. Folic acid can help to prevent neural-tube birth defects.
Category: Safe and Effective Care Environment: Safety and Infection Control
Subcategory: Maternal Infant: Antepartum

46. **a.** The anterior portion of the right leg equals 9% and the anterior plus posterior portions of the right arm equal 9% for a total of 18%. Choices **b**, **c**, and **d** are incorrect.
Category: Physiological Integrity: Physiological Adaptation
Subcategory: Adult: Integumentary Disorders

47. **c.** Parenteral iron is given by intramuscular route using the Z-track technique, which will decrease pain and tracking of the medication during needle withdrawal. Choice **a** is incorrect. Proper technique includes changing the needle after drawing up the medication and before administering the injection to prevent staining of the skin. Choice **b** is incorrect. The site should not be massaged after the injection, because massaging the area may result in staining of the skin. Choice **d** is incorrect. An air lock should be used, but the Z-track method will prevent pain.
Category: Safe and Effective Care Environment: Safety and Infection Control
Subcategory: Adult: Hematological Disorders

48. **b.** In general, an LPN or LVN can perform the same tasks as a nursing assistant (e.g., skin care, range of motion exercises, ambulation, grooming, and hygiene measures) in addition to dressing changes, endotracheal suctioning (1); medication administration (oral, intramuscular, and subcutaneous) (4 and 5); and urinary catheterization (6). Choices **a**, **c**, and **d** are incorrect. Client admission assessments (2) and administration of intravenous medications (3) are the responsibility of the registered nurse.
Category: Safe and Effective Care Environment: Management of Care
Subcategory: Adult: Miscellaneous

49. **a.** The DTaP vaccine, which includes diphtheria, tetanus, and pertussis, is usually one of the vaccinations given at the two-month well child exam. Choice **b** is incorrect. The influenza vaccination should not be administered to children less than six months of age. Choice **c** is incorrect. The MMR vaccine, which includes measles, mumps, and rubella, should not be administered to children less than 12 months of age. Choice **d** is incorrect. The varicella vaccination should not be administered to children less than 12 months of age.
Category: Physiological Integrity: Reduction of Risk Potential
Subcategory: Pediatrics: Assessment

50. **c.** Establishing a relaxing prebed routine will provide signals for the client's body that it is time for sleep, and thus will promote sleep. Choice **a** is incorrect. Amitriptyline, while having the side effect of drowsiness, is used for the treatment of depression, not to help clients sleep. Choice **b** is incorrect. Watching television is considered to be a stimulating activity and is therefore contraindicated for promoting sleep. Choice **d** is incorrect. Sitting in the room with the client may distract the client from sleeping and will reward the client for not sleeping.
Category: Health Promotion and Maintenance
Subcategory: Mental Health: Cognitive Disorders

51. **d.** Preterm labor occurs between 27 and 36 weeks of pregnancy. Symptoms include regular contractions occurring at least every 10 minutes that are not relieved with position changes. Cervical dilation is also a symptom of preterm labor. Choice **a** is incorrect. Symptoms of cervical incompetence include cervical dilation but not regular contractions. Choice **b** is incorrect. Symptoms of placenta previa include painless vaginal bleeding but not cervical dilation or contractions. Choice **c** is incorrect. A symptom of preeclampsia includes elevated blood pressure.
Category: Physiological Integrity: Physiological Adaptation
Subcategory: Maternal Infant: Maternal Complications: Antepartum

52. **d.** Potassium chloride is never given by bolus (IV push). Administering potassium chloride by IV push can result in cardiac arrest. Choice **a** is incorrect. When administrating potassium chloride intravenously, it must always be diluted in fluid. Normal saline is recommended. Dextrose solution is avoided because this type of solution increases intracellular potassium. The IV site is monitored closely because potassium chloride can irritate the veins and phlebitis can occur. Choice **b** is incorrect. The nurse should monitor the client's urine output during potassium chloride administration and must notify the physician if the urine output falls below 30 mL per hour. Choice **c** is incorrect. Potassium chloride is always administered via an electronic IV pump or controller.
Category: Physiological Integrity: Pharmacological and Parenteral Therapies
Subcategory: Adult: Miscellaneous

53. **d.** Varicose veins are more common after the age of 30, especially in clients whose occupations require prolonged standing. They also occur more frequently in pregnant women and those with a positive family history of varicose veins and systemic problems such as heart disease. Another risk factor is obesity. Choices **a**, **b**, and **c** are incorrect. There is no information in this client profile to indicate these conditions.
Category: Health Promotion and Maintenance
Subcategory: Adult: Cardiovascular Disorders

54. **a.** Arranging for an interpreter would be the best practice when communicating with a client who speaks a different language. Choice **b** is incorrect. Speaking loudly when communicating with a client is inappropriate and an ineffective way to communicate. Choice **c** is incorrect. Speaking to a client only when the family is present is inappropriate because it violates privacy; additionally, it is not certain that information will be correctly translated. Choice **d** is incorrect. Standing close to a client and speaking loudly during interactions is an inappropriate and ineffective way to communicate.
Category: Psychosocial Integrity
Subcategory: Adult: Miscellaneous

55. **a.** The woman is most likely experiencing an amniotic fluid embolism and should be positioned in the left lateral position to facilitate maternal and fetal circulation and oxygenation. Choice **b** is incorrect. While the right lateral position might be considered, the left lateral position is a better choice because oxygenation to both the mother and the fetus is facilitated. Choice **c** is incorrect. Semi-Fowler's position is when the client lies supine with the head of the bed elevated 30 degrees. Clients receiving tubing feedings are placed in the semi-Fowler's position. Choice **d** is incorrect. The Trendelenburg position is when the client's head is tilted down; it is used for treatment of hemodynamic shock. It would not be used in this scenario because increased blood flow is needed for both the mother and the fetus, which is best accomplished through the left lateral position.
Category: Physiological Integrity: Reduction of Risk Potential
Subcategory: Maternal Infant: Intrapartum

56. c. Troponin is a regulatory protein found in striated muscle. Troponins function together in the contractile apparatus for striated muscles and skeletal muscles in the myocardium. Increased amounts of troponins are released into the bloodstream when an infarction occurs, causing damage to the myocardium. A troponin-T value that is higher than 0.2 ng/mL is consistent with a myocardial infarction. Choice **a** is incorrect. A normal serum troponin-T level is 0.0 to 0.2 ng/mL. Choice **b** is incorrect. A normal serum troponin-T level is lower than 0.2 ng/mL. A level of 0.7 ng/mL is not indicative of angina but rather a myocardial infarction. Choice **d** is incorrect. An elevated troponin level is not associated with gastritis. Gastritis can be confused with chest pain associated with a myocardial infarction.
Category: Physiological Integrity: Physiological Adaptation
Subcategory: Adult: Cardiovascular Disorders

57. b. The inactivated polio virus is not recommended at this time, unless the child is behind on her inactivated polio immunizations. Choice **a** is incorrect. The CDC recommends that children receive the HPV (human papillomavirus) vaccine between the ages of 11 and 12. Choice **c** is incorrect. The CDC recommends yearly influenza vaccinations. Choice **d** is incorrect. The CDC recommends that children receive the meningococcal conjugate vaccine (MCV4) between the ages of 11 and 12.
Category: Physiological Integrity: Reduction of Risk Potential
Subcategory: Pediatrics: Assessment

58. c. The nurse must report situations not only of elder abuse but also child abuse, gunshot wounds, criminal acts, and certain infectious diseases. The client should be told that her information is kept confidential unless it places the nurse under a legal obligation to report the information to the proper authorities. Choices **a** and **b** are incorrect. These options do not address the legal implications of the situation and do not ensure a safe environment for the client. Choice **d** is incorrect. This option does not address the legal implications of the situation and does not ensure a safe environment for the client. Confidential issues are not to be discussed with nonmedical personnel or the client's family or friends without the client's permission.
Category: Safe and Effective Care Environment: Management of Care
Subcategory: Adult: Miscellaneous

59. b. Establishing a client food contract (2) will help the client to control binging, and staying with the client for two hours after eating (3) will help prevent opportunities for the client to purge. Choice **a** is incorrect. Establishing a client food contract (2) will help the client to control binging, but the client should be provided with nutrient-dense, not calorie-dense foods (1). Choice **c** is incorrect. Staying with the client for two hours after eating (3) will help prevent opportunities for the client to purge, but limiting time in the bathroom (4) will not. Choice **d** is incorrect. The client should be provided nutrient-dense, not calorie-dense foods (1). Limiting time in the bathroom (4) will not prevent opportunities for the client to purge after eating.
Category: Safe and Effective Care Environment: Management of Care
Subcategory: Mental Health: Eating Disorders

60. d. A potassium level lower than 3.5 mEq/L indicates hypokalemia. Hypokalemia can be a life-threatening occurrence. Specific electrocardiogram changes indicative of hypokalemia include inverted T-waves, ST-segment depression, and prominent U-waves. Choice **a** is incorrect. In hypokalemia, which is indicated by the client's potassium level, the P waves are not affected. Absent P-waves are associated with atrial fibrillation. Choice **b** is incorrect. In hypokalemia, which is indicated by the client's potassium level, there would be depressed ST-segments. Choice **c** is incorrect. In hypokalemia, which is indicated by the client's potassium level, the T waves would be inverted.
Category: Physiological Integrity: Physiological Adaptation
Subcategory: Adult: Electrolyte Imbalances

61. b. The therapeutic range for serum dilantin level is 10 to 20 μg/mL. If the level is below the therapeutic range, the client would experience seizure activity. If the level is too high, the client will be at risk for toxicity. Choices **a**, **c**, and **d** are incorrect. The therapeutic range for serum dilantin level is 10 to 20 μg/mL.
Category: Physiological Integrity: Physiological Adaptation
Subcategory: Adult: Neurological Disorders

62. a. The circumcision site should be assessed for signs of bleeding and for signs of infection. Choice **b** is incorrect. Cleansing the site with a baby wipe is not recommended due to the alcohol content in baby wipes. Choice **c** is incorrect. An infant with a petroleum dressing should not be placed in a radiant warmer due to the risk for burns. Choice **d** is incorrect. The infant's diaper should be secured loosely and changed every four hours. Securing the diaper tightly will cause discomfort.
Category: Safe and Effective Care Environment: Safety and Infection Control
Subcategory: Maternal Infant: Neonate

63. b. NPH insulin is an intermediate-acting insulin. It peaks in 6 to 12 hours after administration. Its onset is 1 to 2 hours, and its duration is 18 to 24 hours. In this scenario, the medication was given at 7 a.m.; therefore, the nurse should monitor for hypoglycemia during the peak action of the medication, which would be between 1 p.m. and 7 p.m. Choices **a**, **c**, and **d** are incorrect. NPH insulin peaks in 6 to 12 hours after administration.
Category: Physiological Integrity: Physiological Adaptation
Subcategory: Adult: Endocrine Disorders

64. c. Eye prophylaxis in newborns is for the prevention of eye infections caused by gonorrhea and/or trichomoniasis infection. Choice **a** is incorrect. Candidiasis or yeast infections are not passed from mother to fetus during the delivery process. Choice **b** is incorrect. Prevention of transmission of active genital herpes from mother to fetus is accomplished through cesarean section. Choice **d** is incorrect. Prevention of transmission of B strep from mother to fetus is accomplished through administration of IV antibiotics to the mother just prior to the delivery.
Category: Safe and Effective Care Management: Safety and Infection Control
Subcategory: Maternal Infant: Neonate Medications

65. c. The nurse will ask the client to take a deep breath, hold it, and bear down during the tubing change. Called the Valsalva maneuver, this step helps avoid air embolus during tubing changes. Choices **a** and **b** are incorrect. These actions are inappropriate and could potentially cause an air embolism during the tubing change. Choice **d** is incorrect. If the center venous line is located on the right side, the client should be instructed to turn his or her head to the left, not the right. In this situation, turning the head to the right will increase intrathoracic pressure.
Category: Physiological Integrity: Pharmacological and Parenteral Therapies
Subcategory: Adult: Endocrine Disorders

66. c. The child with congestive heart failure should be offered small meals frequently. Choice **a** is incorrect. Morphine sulfate is administered for pain. There is no indication that this child is in pain. Choice **b** is incorrect. Due to fluid in the lungs, the child will most likely not tolerate the head of the bed being lowered. Choice **d** is incorrect. The environment should be kept nonstimulating for a child admitted with congestive heart failure.
Category: Safe and Effective Care Environment: Management of Care
Subcategory: Pediatrics: Cardiovascular Disorders

67. c. The V6 lead is placed at the fifth intercostal space at the midaxillary line (area 3). Correct placement of the leads is essential when performing a 12-lead ECG to accurately document the electrical potential of the heart. V6 is one of the precordial leads and, in combination with the other leads, records potential in the horizontal plane. Choices **a**, **b**, and **d** are incorrect. The V6 lead is placed at the fifth intercostal space at the midaxillary line (area 3).
Category: Physiological Integrity: Reduction of Risk Potential
Subcategory: Adult: Cardiovascular Disorders

68. a. Impulsiveness occurs during the manic phase of bipolar disorder. Choice **b** is incorrect. Feelings of hopelessness occur during the depressive phase of bipolar disorder. Choice **c** is incorrect. Suicidal thoughts occur during the depressive phase of bipolar disorder. Choice **d** is incorrect. Anxiety is not a symptom of either the manic or the depressive phase of bipolar disorder.
Category: Safe and Effective Care Environment: Safety and Infection Control
Subcategory: Mental Health: Mood Disorders

69. d. To determine whether costovertebral tenderness (a sign of glomerulonephritis) is present, the nurse should percuss the costovertebral angle, that is, the angle over each kidney that's formed by the lateral and downward curve of the lowest rib and the vertebral column. The costovertebral angle can be percussed by placing the palm of one hand over the costovertebral angle and striking it with the fist of the other hand. Choices **a**, **b**, and **c** are incorrect. The physical examination revealed right-sided costovertebral tenderness. The areas indicated in these choices are incorrect.
Category: Physiological Integrity: Physiological Adaptation
Subcategory: Adult: Renal Disorders

70. d. The nursing educator should stop the nurse from unclamping the cord and remind the nurse that the clamp should not be removed for the first 24 hours after birth. Choice **a** is incorrect. The cord should not be unclamped for the first 24 hours after birth, so the baby does not need to be distracted. Choice **b** is incorrect. While it is true that the cord will shrivel and fall off within 7 to 10 days, the clamp should not be removed for the first 24 hours after birth. Choice **c** is incorrect. The nurse should not be encouraged to continue, as the cord should not be unclamped for the first 24 hours after birth.
Category: Safe and Effective Care Management: Safety and Infection Control
Subcategory: Maternal Infant: Neonate Care

71. a. Violations of confidentiality occur when client information is discussed with nonmedical persons, such as family or friends, without the client's permission. Choices **b**, **c**, and **d** are incorrect. It is appropriate to discuss a client's diagnosis with other members of the healthcare team.
Category: Safe and Effective Care Environment: Management of Care
Subcategory: Adult: Musculoskeletal Disorders

72. c. When a chest tube is removed, the client is instructed to perform the Valsalva maneuver (which is to bear down). The physician then quickly withdraws the chest tube and, with the assistance of the nurse, applies an airtight dressing to the site. Alternatively, the client can also be instructed to take a deep breath and hold the breath while the tube is removed. Choices **a**, **b**, and **d** are incorrect. It would be inappropriate as well as inaccurate to instruct the client to follow any of these instructions during chest tube removal.
Category: Safe and Effective Care Environment: Safety and Infection Control
Subcategory: Adult: Cardiovascular Disorders

73. a. The nurse should instruct the client to first exhale fully (step 1). The client should then place the mouthpiece of the spirometer in the mouth, inhale, and hold the breath for three seconds (step 2). The client should then exhale passively (step 3). Finally, the client should take a deep breath and cough (step 4). Choices **b**, **c**, and **d** are incorrect.
Category: Safe and Effective Care Environment: Management of Care
Subcategory: Adult: Respiratory Disorders

74. b. A child with aortic stenosis typically will not present with cyanosis. Choices **a**, **c**, and **d** are incorrect. Each of these conditions is a symptom of aortic stenosis.
Category: Physiological Integrity: Physiological Adaptation
Subcategory: Pediatrics: Cardiovascular Disorders

75. c. Finger foods should be offered frequently to the client with severe depression who exhibits a loss of appetite and lack of interest in food, because smaller portions will likely be less disagreeable. Choice **a** is incorrect. Experiencing a decreased appetite and a loss of interest in food is a symptom of the depression; therefore the client will not want to select his or her own food. Choice **b** is incorrect. Although an attractive presentation of food is important for the client, the client with severe depression who exhibits a loss of appetite and lack of interest in food will not want to eat large meals. Choice **d** is incorrect. To ensure the intake of adequate nutrients, nutrient-dense versus calorie-dense foods should be offered to the client with severe depression who exhibits a loss of appetite and lack of interest in food.
Category: Physiological Integrity: Basic Care and Comfort
Subcategory: Mental Health: Mood Disorders

76. b. Lanugo develops during the fifth month of gestation. It is common for neonates to have lanugo, and it will generally disappear on its own. Choice **a** is incorrect. The nurse should recognize the fine downy hair as lanugo, a common occurrence in newborns. Choice **c** is incorrect. Milia appear as small white bumps over the infant's nose, chin, and/or cheeks. Choice **d** is incorrect. Lanugo will generally disappear on its own.
Category: Psychosocial Integrity
Subcategory: Maternal Infant: Neonate Assessment

77. d. Oliguria, or a low urine output, occurs during cardiogenic shock due to reduced blood flow to the kidneys. Other typical signs of cardiogenic shock include low blood pressure, rapid and weak pulse, and signs of diminished blood flow to the brain (confusion and restlessness). Cardiogenic shock is a serious complication of a myocardial infarction, often with mortality rates approaching 90%. Choice **a** is incorrect. The client would experience a rapid and weak pulse, not bradycardia, which is a slow pulse. Choice **b** is incorrect. The client would experience a decreased blood pressure, not an elevated blood pressure. Choice **c** is incorrect. Fever is not a sign or symptom associated with cardiogenic shock.
Category: Physiological Integrity: Reduction of Risk Potential
Subcategory: Adult: Cardiovascular Disorders

78. **a.** The use of Pitocin to induce labor places the client at risk for postpartum hemorrhage from the uterus's becoming soft or boggy when the Pitocin wears off. Choices **b, c,** and **d** are incorrect. The use of Pitocin to induce labor does not increase the risk for any of these conditions in the postpartum period.
Category: Physiological Integrity: Pharmacological and Parenteral Therapies
Subcategory: Maternal Infant: Maternal Medications

79. **d.** First, the nurse will need to calculate the number of milligrams per milliliter:
$\frac{50 \text{ mg}}{250 \text{ mL}} = \frac{1 \text{ mg}}{5 \text{ mL}} = \frac{0.2 \text{ mg}}{1 \text{ mL}}$
Next, the nurse will need to calculate the number of micrograms in each milligram: $0.2 \text{ mg} \times 1{,}000 \text{ mcg} = 200 \text{ mcg}$.
Choices **a, b,** and **c** are incorrect.
Category: Physiological Integrity: Pharmacological and Parenteral Therapies
Subcategory: Adult: Cardiovascular Disorders

80. **a.** Eating dry crackers before getting out of bed in the morning can decrease feelings of morning sickness. Choice **b** is incorrect. The client should eat small, frequent meals throughout the day. Choice **c** is incorrect. Foods high in fat can increase feelings of morning sickness. Choice **d** is incorrect. The client should increase fluids between meals, not during meals.
Category: Physiological Integrity: Basic Care and Comfort
Subcategory: Maternal Infant: Antepartum

81. **b.** The client should maintain the head of the bed between 15 and 30 degrees (1). Monitoring neurological status using the GCS is correct (3). An ICP greater than 20 mm Hg indicates increased ICP, and the nurse should notify the healthcare provider immediately if this occurs (4). Choices **a, c,** and **d** are incorrect. The nurse should not encourage the client to cough (2) nor engage in range-of-motion exercises (5), as these will increase ICP and should be avoided in the early postoperative stages.
Category: Physiological Integrity: Physiological Adaptation
Subcategory: Adult: Neurological Disorders

82. **d.** The first sign of Parkinson's disease is usually tremors. The client is often the first to notice the tremors. Tremors may initially be minimal. Choice **a** is incorrect. Akinesia, the inability to initiate movement, is a later sign of Parkinson's disease. It follows bradykinesia. Choice **b** is incorrect. Bradykinesia, the slowness of movement, is the third sign generally associated with Parkinson's disease. Choice **c** is incorrect. Rigidity is the second sign generally associated with Parkinson's disease.
Category: Physiological Integrity: Physiological Adaptation
Subcategory: Adult: Neurological Disorders

83. c. One of the symptoms of rheumatic fever is painful joints. Choice **a** is incorrect. The sedimentation rate would be increased with rheumatic fever. Choice **b** is incorrect. Rheumatic fever occurs after a partially or untreated streptococcal throat infection. Choice **d** is incorrect. While one of the symptoms of rheumatic fever is shortness of breath, this is not typically accompanied by inspiratory pain.
Category: Physiological Integrity: Physiological Adaptation
Subcategory: Pediatrics: Cardiovascular Disorders

84. b. Chest physiotherapy is best performed before meals to avoid tiring the client or inducing vomiting. Choice **a** is incorrect. Chest physiotherapy performed after meals risks tiring the client or inducing vomiting. Choice **c** is incorrect. Scheduling chest physiotherapy around the client's convenience is inappropriate. Choice **d** is incorrect. Scheduling chest physiotherapy around the nurse's convenience is inappropriate.
Category: Safe and Effective Care Environment: Safety and Infection Control
Subcategory: Adult: Respiratory Disorders

85. b. As the depressed client begins to have increased energy levels, the risk for suicide increases. Choice **a** is incorrect. While allowing the depressed client to verbalize feelings is important, as the depressed client begins to have increased energy levels, the risk for suicide increases and assumes a higher priority than verbalization of feelings. Choice **c** is incorrect. Although ensuring adequate nutritional intake is important, assessing for suicide risk is a higher priority, especially as the depressed client begins to have increased energy levels. Choice **d** is incorrect. Clients taking monoamine oxidase inhibitors as treatment for depression are at risk for a hypertensive crisis. However, Celexa is not a monoamine oxidase inhibitor; therefore, while monitoring this client's blood pressure is important, it is a lower priority than assessing for thoughts of suicide.
Category: Safe and Effective Care Management: Safety and Infection Control
Subcategory: Mental Health: Mood Disorders

86. b. Cracked nipples are often caused by having only the nipple versus the nipple and areola inserted into the infant's mouth, causing incorrect latching. Choice **a** is incorrect. Cracked nipples can be prevented by having the infant latch on correctly. Choice **c** is incorrect. The nipple and the areola should be guided into the infant's mouth. Choice **d** is incorrect. The nipples should not be washed with soap, because soap can cause the skin to dry and crack.
Category: Physiological Integrity: Basic Care and Comfort
Subcategory: Maternal Infant: Maternal Complications: Postpartum

87. b. Decorticate posturing is also called decorticate response, decorticate rigidity, flexor posturing, or, colloquially, mummy baby. Clients with decorticate posturing present with the arms flexed, or bent inward on the chest, the hands clenched into fists, and the legs extended and feet turned inward. A person displaying decorticate posturing in response to pain gets a score of 3 in the motor section of the Glasgow Coma Scale. Choice **a** is incorrect. Decerebrate posturing—also called decerebrate response, decerebrate rigidity, or extensor posturing—is the involuntary extension of the upper extremities in response to external stimuli. In decerebrate posturing, the head is arched back, the arms are extended by the sides, and the legs are extended. Choice **c** is incorrect. Opisthotonus is a state of a severe hyperextension and spasticity in which an individual's head, neck, and spinal column enter into a complete "bridging" or arching position. This abnormal posturing—an extrapyramidal effect—is caused by spasms of the axial muscles along the spinal column. Choice **d** is incorrect. In anatomy, the prone position is a position of the body lying face down. In anatomical terminology, the ventral side is down, and the dorsal side is up. The prone position is the opposite of the supine position, which is face up.
Category: Physiological Integrity: Physiological Adaptation
Subcategory: Adult: Neurological Disorders

88. b. Clients with gout should avoid foods that are high in purines, such as cod (2), liver (5), and sardines (6), as well as anchovies, kidneys, sweetbreads, lentils, and alcoholic beverages—especially beer and wine. Choices **a**, **c**, and **d** are incorrect. Chocolate (1), eggs (3), and green, leafy vegetables (4) aren't high in purines and are acceptable foods for the client to eat.
Category: Physiological Integrity: Basic Care and Comfort
Subcategory: Adult: Musculoskeletal Disorders

89. a. The infant with an Apgar score of 4 to 7, while not needing resuscitation measures, may benefit from gentle stimulation and the administration of oxygen. Choice **b** is incorrect. Apgar scores of 0 to 3 require resuscitation measures. Choice **c** is incorrect. Infants with an Apgar score of 4 to 7 may benefit from gentle stimulation and the administration of oxygen. It would be inappropriate to complete the first bath at this time. Choice **d** is incorrect. While bonding is important, this infant is in need of gentle stimulation and administration of oxygen.
Category: Safe and Effective Care Environment: Management of Care
Subcategory: Maternal Infant: Neonate Assessment

90. **b.** The axillary (1) and tympanic (3) routes are the preferred methods for taking the temperature of a three-year-old. Choice **a** is incorrect. It is difficult to obtain an accurate oral temperature (2) on a three-year-old. Choice **c** is incorrect. It is not appropriate to take a rectal temperature (4) on a three-year-old due to the risk of perforating the anus. Choice **d** is incorrect. It is difficult to obtain an accurate oral temperature (2) on a three-year-old. It is not appropriate to take a rectal temperature (4) on a three-year-old due to the risk of perforating the anus.
Category: Safe and Effective Care Environment: Safety and Infection Control
Subcategory: Pediatrics:

91. **d.** Mafenide acetate (Sulfamylon) is bacteriostatic for gram-negative and gram-positive organisms and is used to treat burns to reduce bacteria present in the avascular tissues. The nurse should explain to the client that the medication will cause local discomfort and a burning sensation and that this is a normal reaction. Choice **a** is incorrect. Altering the prescribed amount of medication is not within the scope of practice of the nurse. Choice **b** is incorrect. Discontinuing the medication is not within the scope of practice of the nurse. Choice **c** is incorrect. It is unnecessary to notify the healthcare provider, as this is a normal occurrence when this medication is used.
Category: Physiological Integrity: Pharmacological and Parenteral Therapies
Subcategory: Adult: Integumentary Disorders

92. **a.** The cardinal physiologic abnormalities of acute respiratory failure are hypoventilation, hypoxemia, and hypercapnia. The nurse should focus on resolving these problems. Choices **b**, **c**, and **d** are incorrect. The nurse should not focus on hyperoxemia, hypocapnia, hyperventilation, hypertension, or hypotension. Signs of respiratory failure include hypoventilation, hypoxemia, and hypercapnia.
Category: Physiological Integrity: Physiological Adaptation
Subcategory: Adult: Respiratory Disorders

93. **a.** Graves' disease, or hyperthyroidism, is a hypermetabolic state that is associated with weight loss as well as rapid, bounding pulses (1), heat intolerance (4), tremors (5), and nervousness (6). Choices **b** and **c** are incorrect. Bradycardia (2) and constipation (3) are signs and symptoms of hypothyroidism, not hyperthyroidism. Choice **d** is incorrect. Rapid, bounding pulses (1) and nervousness (6) are other symptoms of Graves' disease.
Category: Health Promotion and Maintenance
Subcategory: Adult: Endocrine Disorders

94. **c.** The nurse should gently massage the fundus to increase its tone. Choice **a** is incorrect. While it is appropriate for the nurse to document the finding of a boggy fundus, the nurse should first massage the fundus to prevent postpartum hemorrhage. Choice **b** is incorrect. Voiding will not change the tone of the fundus. Choice **d** is incorrect. The nurse should first gently massage the fundus to increase its tone. If the fundus remains boggy, the physician should then be notified.
Category: Physiological Integrity: Reduction of Risk Potential
Subcategory: Maternal Infant: Maternal Complications: Postpartum

95. b. Clients with antisocial personality disorder are at risk for harming themselves (2) and others (3) and are at risk for developing substance abuse problems (4). Choices **a**, **c**, and **d** are incorrect. Clients with antisocial personality disorder do not exhibit anxiety (1).
Category: Safe and Effective Care Environment: Safety and Infection Control
Subcategory: Mental Health: Personality Disorders

96. a. To test for the Babinski reflex, the nurse uses a tongue blade to slowly stroke the lateral side of the underside of the foot. The nurse will start at the heel and move toward the great toe. The normal response in an adult is plantar flexion of the toes. Upward movement of the great toe and fanning of the little toe, called the Babinski reflex, is abnormal. Choices **b**, **c**, and **d** are incorrect. These locations are incorrect starting points to test the Babinski reflex.
Category: Health Promotion and Maintenance
Subcategory: Adult: Neurological Disorders

97. b. The nurse should elevate the head of the bed, as this will allow for increased lung expansion by decreasing ascites pressing on the diaphragm. Following this intervention, the client requires reassessment. Choice **a** is incorrect. Heart sounds are assessed with a routine physical assessment. Choice **c** is incorrect. There is no indication that blood cultures are needed. Choice **d** is incorrect. A paracentesis is reserved for clients symptomatic of ascites with impaired respiration or abdominal pain not responding to other measures such as sodium restriction and the administration of diuretic medications.
Category: Physiological Integrity: Physiological Adaptation
Subcategory: Adult: Gastrointestinal Disorders

98. a. When a client has eyedrops and eye ointment scheduled at the same time, the nurse should administer the eyedrops first and then the eye ointment. The instillation of two medications is separated by a time period of three to five minutes. Choice **b** is incorrect. This is not the proper technique; it isn't necessary to wait 10 minutes before administering the eye ointment. Choices **c** and **d** are incorrect. These are not the proper techniques; the eyedrops should be administered first.
Category: Physiological Integrity: Pharmacological and Parenteral Therapies
Subcategory: Adult: Eye Disorders

99. b. A prenatal fetal heart rate of 130 beats per minute is within the normal limits of 120 to 160 beats per minute and should be documented as such. Choice **a** is incorrect. A prenatal fetal heart rate of 130 beats per minute is within the normal limits of 120 to 160 beats per minute. This information alone does not precipitate an ultrasound. Choice **c** is incorrect. A prenatal fetal heart rate of 130 beats per minute is within the normal limits of 120 to 160 beats per minute; therefore, the nurse does not need to reassess the rate at this time. Choice **d** is incorrect. A prenatal fetal heart rate of 130 beats per minute is within the normal limits of 120 to 160 beats per minute; therefore, the mother does not need to be positioned on her left side.
Category: Physiological Integrity: Physiological Adaptation
Subcategory: Maternal Infant: Fetal Assessment

100. c. The Guthrie test screens for phenylketonuria. Choice **a** is incorrect. The screening test for cystic fibrosis is the immunoreactive trypsinogen (IRT). Choice **b** is incorrect. The screening test for Down syndrome is the maternal alpha fetoprotein test. Choice **d** is incorrect. The screening test for spina bifida is the maternal alpha fetoprotein test.
Category: Physiological Integrity: Reduction of Risk Potential
Subcategory: Pediatrics: Endocrine Disorders

101. c. This medication will not stain the client's skin. Choice **a** is incorrect. This medication is an antibacterial, which has a broad spectrum of activity against gram-negative bacteria, gram-positive bacteria, and yeast. Choice **b** is incorrect. This medication is directly applied to the wounds. Choice **d** is incorrect. This medication will help heal the client's burned areas.
Category: Physiological Integrity: Pharmacological and Parenteral Therapies
Subcategory: Adult: Integumentary Disorders

102. a. Following glaucoma surgery, clients will use miotic eyedrops. These agents cause the pupil to constrict, which can compromise a client's ability to adjust safely to night vision. For safety, extra lighting should be added to the home. Choice **b** is incorrect. It is unnecessary for the client to decrease fluid intake. This intervention is not associated with glaucoma surgery. Choice **c** is incorrect. The client is not restricted from exercise; however, excessive exertion should be avoided. Choice **d** is incorrect. There is no need to avoid sunlight by wearing dark sunglasses. Sunlight will not disturb the client's eyesight.
Category: Physiological Integrity: Basic Care and Comfort
Subcategory: Adult: Eye Disorders

103. d. Echopraxia is imitation of another's movements. Choice **a** is incorrect. Aphasia is the inability to use and/or understand language. Choice **b** is incorrect. Ataxia is a lack of coordination when performing voluntary muscle movements. Choice **c** is incorrect. Echolalia is repetition of a word or phrase.
Category: Psychosocial Integrity
Subcategory: Mental Health: Schizophrenic Disorders

104. a. When the fetal head is palpated at the top of the fundus (position 4), the fetus is in a breech presentation. Choices **b** and **c** are incorrect. When the fetus is lying horizontally across the fundus, it is referred to as being in a transverse presentation and the fetal head would be palpated at the side of the abdomen, such as in position 2 or position 3. Choice **d** is incorrect. The vertex presentation occurs when the fetus is in a head-down position. If the fetus were in the vertex presentation, the fetal head would be palpated at position 1.
Category: Physiological Integrity: Physiological Adaptation
Subcategory: Maternal Infant: Fetal Assessment

105. c. Essential hypertension (also called primary hypertension) is defined as a consistent systolic blood pressure level greater than 140 mm Hg and a consistent diastolic blood pressure level greater than 90 mm Hg. Choices **a**, **b**, and **d** are incorrect. These blood pressure readings are not the defined values for essential hypertension.
Category: Physiological Integrity: Reduction of Risk Potential
Subcategory: Adult: Cardiovascular Disorders

106. c. Arterial steal syndrome may be experienced by clients with renal failure after the creation of a fistula. Such clients often exhibit pallor and diminished pulse resulting from the fistula. Additionally, the client may also complain of pain distal to the fistula. The pain is caused by tissue ischemia. Choice **a** is incorrect. Edema is not a sign or symptom of arterial steal syndrome. Choice **b** is incorrect. Edema and reddish discoloration are not signs or symptoms of arterial steal syndrome. Choice **d** is incorrect. Warmth and redness may be indicative of an infection, not arterial steal syndrome.
Category: Physiological Integrity: Physiological Adaptation
Subcategory: Adult: Renal Disorders

107. d. This action shows acceptance of the change in body image. By touching the altered body part, the client recognizes the body change and establishes that the change is real. Choice **a** is incorrect. When the client avoids openly and readily speaking about the surgery, this reflects some level of denial, instead of full acceptance of the change. Choice **b** is incorrect. Requesting the spouse to leave the room reflects denial, not acceptance, of the change. It also signifies that the client is ashamed of the change and is not coping with it. Choice **c** is incorrect. In closing his eyes when the colostomy is exposed, the client reflects denial, not acceptance, of the change.
Category: Psychosocial Integrity
Subcategory: Adult: Gastrointestinal Disorders

108. d. By reflecting back the father's thoughts, this statement encourages the father to continue to verbalize his feelings and concerns. Choice **a** is incorrect. While home care will usually be ordered for children with new ostomies, the nurse should encourage the father to verbalize his feelings and concerns. Choice **b** is incorrect. This statement disregards the father's fears and concerns, and discourages the father from further verbalization of his feelings and concerns. Choice **c** is incorrect. While the procedure may not be difficult, this statement disregards the father's feelings and concerns, and discourages the father from further verbalization of his feelings and concerns.
Category: Psychosocial Integrity
Subcategory: Pediatrics: Gastrointestinal Disorders

109. c. The nurse correctly identifies this rhythm as sinus rhythm with premature ventricular contractions. PVCs are extra, abnormal heartbeats that begin in one of the heart's two lower pumping chambers (ventricles). These extra beats disrupt the regular heart rhythm. Unifocal PVCs look alike; if they differed in appearance, they would be called multifocal PVCs, as seen in this tracing. Choice **a** is incorrect. This tracing does not indicate sinus rhythm with premature atrial contractions. PACs can momentarily interrupt normal sinus rhythm by inserting an extra heartbeat. PACs are caused by occasional, early (or premature) electrical impulses that can arise from almost anywhere within the cardiac atria. In other words, PACs are early atrial heartbeats that are not produced by the sinus node. Choice **b** is incorrect. This tracing does not indicate sinus rhythm with second-degree AV block—Mobitz I. Mobitz type-I AV block shows a progressive PR interval prolongation preceding a nonconducted P-wave. Choice **d** is incorrect. This tracing does not indicate ventricular pacing. Ventricular pacing with 100% capture is diagnosed when the electrocardiogram shows only complexes that result from the ventricular pacemaker; each QRS complex is preceded by a pacemaker stimulus/pacer spike.
Category: Physiological Integrity: Physiological Adaptation
Subcategory: Adult: Cardiovascular Disorders

110. d. Symptoms of ectopic pregnancy include amenorrhea, slight vaginal bleeding, and unilateral pelvic pain. Choice **a** is incorrect. Cervical dilation at five weeks gestation places the client at risk for spontaneous abortion. Choice **b** is incorrect. The nurse would expect to find a small amount of vaginal bleeding, not a hemorrhage, in the client with an ectopic pregnancy. Choice **c** is incorrect. Nausea and vomiting during early pregnancy might be indicative of morning sickness or hyperemesis gravidarum.
Category: Physiological Integrity: Physiological Adaptation
Subcategory: Maternal Infant: Maternal Complications: Antepartum

111. d. Stadol is an opioid administered for pain relief during labor. Adverse reactions include respiratory depression; therefore, it should not be given if the maternal respiratory rate is less than 12 breaths per minute. Choice **a** is incorrect. Stadol is an opioid administered for pain relief during labor. The fundal height does not influence the nurse's decision to administer or to hold Stadol. Choice **b** is incorrect. Stadol does not adversely impact the maternal heart rate. Choice **c** is incorrect. Lochia refers to the vaginal discharge after labor.
Category: Physiological Integrity: Pharmacological and Parenteral Therapies
Subcategory: Maternal Infant: Maternal Medications

112. d. The nurse should implement interventions to decrease the discomfort of pruritus. This will include those that prevent vasodilation, decrease anxiety, and maintain skin integrity and hydration. Medicated baths with salicylic acid or colloidal oatmeal can be soothing as a temporary relief measure. Choice **a** is incorrect. Administration of antihistamines should be used cautiously, depending on the cause of the pruritus. Choice **b** is incorrect. Administration of topical steroids should be used cautiously, depending on the cause of the pruritus. Choice **c** is incorrect. The use of silk sheets is not a common practice for patients who are hospitalized and experiencing pruritus.
Category: Physiological Integrity: Basic Care and Comfort
Subcategory: Adult: Oncology Disorders

113. c. La belle indifference is a lack of appropriate concern for symptoms and a lack of anxiety that can occur with conversion disorders. Choice **a** is incorrect. Catatonic excitement is excessive motor activity that can occur in catatonic schizophrenia. Choice **b** is incorrect. Catatonic stupor is when a client is in a vegetative-like condition. It occurs with catatonic schizophrenia. Choice **d** is incorrect. Pseudoneurologic manifestation is the term used for conversion disorders where symptoms present and resolve themselves based on the presence of life-stress triggers.
Category: Psychosocial Integrity
Subcategory: Mental Health: Somatoform Disorders

114. b. Skin testing is based on the antigen/antibody response and will show a positive reaction after a client has been exposed to tuberculosis and has formed antibodies to the tuberculosis bacteria. Thus, a positive Mantoux test indicates the production of an immune response. Choices **a**, **c**, and **d** are incorrect. A positive test doesn't confirm that a person is actively immune to tuberculosis or that a person has or will develop tuberculosis. It only confirms exposure to tuberculosis, and exposure doesn't confer immunity.
Category: Safe and Effective Care Environment: Safety and Infection Control
Subcategory: Adult: Respiratory Disorders

115. a. The nurse should provide the mother with an opportunity to hold the infant. This will allow the mother to bond with and grieve for the loss of the child. Choice **b** is incorrect. While labor and delivery units will often utilize a sign or symbol to alert healthcare personnel of the fetal demise, the first action of the nurse should be to provide the mother with an opportunity to hold the infant. Choice **c** is incorrect. It is inappropriate to remove the infant from the room without providing the mother with an opportunity to hold the infant. Choice **d** is incorrect. While referring the mother to a support group is an appropriate measure, it is inappropriate to do so immediately after the delivery.
Category: Psychosocial Integrity
Subcategory: Maternal Infant: Maternal Complications: Intrapartum

116. b. Pain disorder is a type of somatoform disorder where the pain is due to a medical condition that is significant enough to warrant clinical attention; however, psychological factors impact the onset, severity, exacerbation, and/or continuation of the pain. Choice **a** is incorrect. Hypochondria is a somatoform disorder where physical complaints are exaggerated to the point that the client experiences impairment in social or occupational functioning. Choice **c** is incorrect. In a conversion disorder, the client experiences motor/sensory symptoms that are suggestive of a neurological condition, as the anxiety is unconsciously converted into functional defects. Choice **d** is incorrect. In body dysmorphic disorder, there is a pervasive feeling of ugliness due to an imagined or exaggerated physical defect.
Category: Psychosocial Integrity
Subcategory: Mental Health: Somatoform Disorders

117. b. In a female client, the nurse should advance an indwelling urinary catheter two to three inches (5 to 7.5 cm) into the urethra. In a male client, the nurse should advance the catheter six to eight inches. Choices **a**, **c**, and **d** are incorrect. The urinary catheter should be advanced two to three inches (5 to 7.5 cm) into the urethra.
Category: Safe and Effective Care Environment: Safety and Infection Control
Subcategory: Adult: Fluid and Electrolyte Disorders

118. b. The nurse can best palpate the liver by standing on the client's right side and placing his right hand on the client's abdomen, to the right of the midline (area 2). He should point the fingers of his right hand toward the client's head, just under the right rib margin. Choice **a** is incorrect. Area 1 is incorrect placement to palpate the liver, as it is too low. Choice **c** is incorrect. Area 3 is incorrect placement to palpate the liver, as it is on the client's left side. Choice **d** is incorrect. Area 4 is incorrect placement to palpate the liver, as it is too low and on the client's left side.
Category: Health Promotion and Maintenance
Subcategory: Adult: Gastrointestinal Disorders

119. d. The nurse should include instructions for proper hand washing technique, as pinworms are spread when someone with pinworms scratches around the anus, gets the eggs on his or her hands, and then touches a surface or handles food that is later touched or eaten by another person. Choice **a** is incorrect. Tinidazole (Tindamax) is utilized to treat giardiasis. Choice **b** is incorrect. Abdominal cramping is not a symptom of pinworms; it is a symptom of giardiasis. Choice **c** is incorrect. Dehydration is not a symptom of pinworms; it is a symptom of giardiasis.
Category: Physiological Integrity: Reduction of Risk Potential
Subcategory: Pediatrics: Gastrointestinal Disorders

120. d Hypocalcemia—low calcium level in the blood—is defined as a value below 8.6 mg/dL. An elevated phosphorus level is defined as a value above 4.5 mg/dL. Hypocalcemia is a calcium deficit that causes nerve fiber irritability and repetitive muscle spasms. Signs and symptoms of hypocalcemia include cardiac arrhythmias (1). Clients may begin to experience confusion, depression, and forgetfulness. Additional neurological symptoms include memory loss, hallucinations, disorientation, and drowsiness and lethargy (4), Trousseau sign (6), diarrhea, increased clotting times, anxiety, and irritability. The calcium-phosphorus imbalance leads to brittle bones and pathologic fractures (5). Choice **a** is incorrect because signs and symptoms of hypocalcemia include increased, not decreased, clotting times (3). Choice **b** is incorrect because signs and symptoms of hypocalcemia include diarrhea, not constipation (2), and increased clotting times, not decreased clotting times (3). Choice **c** is incorrect because signs and symptoms of hypocalcemia also include cardiac arrhythmias (1).
Category: Physiological Integrity: Reduction of Risk Potential
Subcategory: Adult: Renal Disorders

121. d. The nurse should instruct the client to be seen by the physician that same day so the client can be evaluated and treated, if needed, for mastitis. Choice **a** is incorrect. The mother may be able to continue to breast-feed the infant, depending on the safety of any medications prescribed during lactation. Choice **b** is incorrect. While the client should be evaluated by a physician, this is not a medical emergency necessitating a visit to the emergency room. Choice **c** is incorrect. Having the client wait until the following week to be seen by a physician is too long a time period. The nurse should instruct the client to be seen by the physician that same day so the client can be evaluated and treated, if needed, for mastitis.
Category: Physiological Integrity: Reduction of Risk Potential
Subcategory: Maternal Infant: Maternal Complications: Postpartum

122. c. Vaginisimus (4), vaginal spasms that interfere with sexual intercourse, may occur in sexual pain disorders. Dyspareunia (2), recurrent genital pain during or after intercourse, may also occur in sexual pain disorder. The nurse should assess for both. Choice **a** is incorrect. Aversion (1) occurs in sexual desire disorders when the client experiences fear, disgust, and/or anxiety when confronted with a sexual opportunity. Choices **b** and **d** are incorrect. Hypoactive desire (3) occurs in sexual desire disorders.
Category: Physiological Integrity: Physiological Adaptation
Subcategory: Mental Health: Sexual Disorders

123. b. The fetal heart rate is able to be heard by Doppler during the third month. Choice **a** is incorrect. The fetal heart rate is not able to be heard by Doppler until the third month. Choices **c** and **d** are incorrect. The fetal heart rate is not able to be heard by stethoscope until the fifth month.
Category: Health Promotion and Maintenance
Subcategory: Maternal Infant: Fetal Development

124. b. The Glasgow Coma Scale assesses the client's level of consciousness by testing and scoring three observations: eye opening, motor response, and verbal stimuli response. Clients are scored on their best responses, and these scores are totaled. The highest score is 15. The highest responses in these three categories are spontaneous eye opening (response 5) for four points; obeying motor commands for six points; and orientation to person, place, and time (response 4) for five points. Choice **a** is incorrect. Incomprehensible verbal response (response 2) is a low score of 2 on the Glasgow Coma Scale, and therefore couldn't contribute to a score of 15. Bradycardia and hypotension (response 1) are not taken into consideration when assessing a patient's Glasgow Coma Scale score. Choice **c** is incorrect. Bradycardia and hypotension (response 1) are not taken into consideration when assessing a patient's Glasgow coma score. Responding to localized pain (response 3) is worth five points out of six on the motor scale, so could not contribute to a maximum score of 15. Choice **d** is incorrect. Incomprehensible verbal response (response 2) is a low score of 2 on the Glasgow Coma Scale, and therefore couldn't contribute to a score of 15. Changes in vital signs and unequal pupil size (response 6) occur with increased intracranial pressure and do indicate neurological compromise; however, these findings are not taken into consideration when assessing a patient's Glasgow coma score. Responding to localized pain (response 3) is worth five points out of six on the motor scale, so could not contribute to a maximum score of 15.
Category: Physiological Integrity: Physiological Adaptation
Subcategory: Adult: Neurological Disorders

125. c. The priority nursing intervention is to dilute the corrosive agent. This can be accomplished with either milk or water. Choice **a** is incorrect. Activated charcoal is administered to decrease the amount of toxic substance absorbed through the gastrointestinal system. However, with corrosive agents such as turpentine, the priority is to dilute the corrosive. Choice **b** is incorrect. Cathartics are utilized to hasten expulsion of the substance. However, with corrosive agents such as turpentine, the priority is to dilute the corrosive. Choice **d** is incorrect. Inducing vomiting is contraindicated with corrosive agents.
Category: Safe and Effective Care Environment: Safety and Infection Control
Subcategory: Pediatrics: Gastrointestinal Disorders

126. b. This tracing is asystole. Asystole (flat line) is a state of no cardiac electrical activity; hence, there are no contractions of the myocardium and no cardiac output or blood flow. Choice **a** is incorrect. This tracing does not show artifact. As a result of artifact, normal components of the ECG are distorted. Choices **c** and **d** are incorrect. This tracing is not coarse or fine ventricular fibrillation (VF). VF is a rhythm in which multiple areas within the ventricles display marked variation in depolarization and repolarization. Since there is no organized ventricular depolarization, the ventricles do not contract as a unit. When observed directly, the ventricular myocardium appears to be quivering. There is no cardiac output. The terms *coarse* and *fine* have been used to describe the amplitude of the waveforms in VF. Coarse VF usually indicates the recent onset of VF, which can be readily corrected by prompt defibrillation. The presence of fine VF that approaches asystole often means there has been a considerable delay since collapse, and successful resuscitation is more difficult.
Category: Physiological Integrity: Physiological Adaptation
Subcategory: Adult: Cardiovascular Disorders

127. c. Complications and/or side effects of the lidocaine infusion include tinnitus, as well as dizziness, blurred vision, tremors, numbness and tingling of extremities, excessive perspiration, hypotension, seizures, and coma. Cardiac effects include slowed conduction and cardiac arrest. Choices **a**, **b**, and **d** are incorrect. These conditions are not considered side effects related to the administration of IV lidocaine.
Category: Physiological Integrity: Pharmacological and Parenteral Therapies
Subcategory: Adult: Cardiovascular Disorders

128. c. The client is most likely experiencing HELLP syndrome (hemolysis, elevated liver enzymes, lower platelet count), which can be a complication of preeclampsia or eclampsia. In patients experiencing HELLP syndrome, a coagulation cascade is activated. This in turn creates fibrin formation in small blood vessels, leading to microangiopathic hemolytic anemia and destruction of red blood cells with consumption of platelets. Palpation of the abdomen is contraindicated at this time due to the potential for liver rupture. Choice **a** is incorrect. Administration of magnesium sulfate per order should be continued to assist in the management of the client's eclampsia. Choice **b** is incorrect. Fetal monitoring should occur to assess fetal well-being. Choice **d** is incorrect. The client is most likely experiencing HELLP syndrome and should be prepared for delivery.
Category: Safe and Effective Care Environment: Management of Care
Subcategory: Maternal Infant: Maternal Complications: Antepartum

129. c. The client should receive recumbent t-PA treatment within three hours after the onset of the stroke to have better outcomes. The time from the onset of a stroke to t-PA treatment is critical. Choice **a** is incorrect. While the nurse should identify which medications the client is taking, it is more important to know the onset time of the stroke to determine the course of action for administering t-PA. Choice **b** is incorrect. A complete health assessment and history is not possible when a client is receiving emergency care. Choice **d** is incorrect. Upcoming surgical procedures may need to be delayed, because the administration of t-PA is the priority.
Category: Physiological Integrity: Reduction of Risk Potential
Subcategory: Adult: Neurological Disorders

130. d. Nuts are a good source of thiamine. Choices **a** and **c** are incorrect. Apples and green beans are good sources of vitamins A and C but not thiamine. Choice **b** is incorrect. Fish is a good source of protein but not thiamine.
Category: Health Promotion and Maintenance
Subcategory: Mental Health: Substance Abuse

131. b. A client with a laryngectomy cannot speak, but still needs to communicate. The nurse should plan to develop an alternative communication method. Choice **a** is incorrect. To prevent injury to the tracheal mucosa, the nurse should deflate the tracheostomy cuff or use the minimal leak technique. Choice **c** is incorrect. Post-laryngectomy, edema interferes with the ability to swallow and necessitates tube (enteral) feedings. Choice **d** is incorrect. To decrease edema, the nurse should place the client in the semi-Fowler's position.
Category: Psychosocial Integrity
Subcategory: Adult: Respiratory Disorders

132. c. This response acknowledges the father's concerns and encourages the father to elaborate on his feelings. Choice **a** is incorrect. This statement is most likely not true and it does not allow the father to discuss his concerns and feelings. Choice **b** is incorrect. This statement evades the question and does not address the father's concerns and feelings. Choice **d** is incorrect. This statement shuts down communication between the father and the nurse and does not allow the father to verbalize his concerns and feelings.
Category: Psychosocial Integrity
Subcategory: Pediatrics: Hematologic and Immune Disorders

133. b. This client is exhibiting symptoms of disseminated intravascular coagulation (DIC) that need to be brought to the immediate attention of the physician. Choice **a** is incorrect. There is no need to monitor the client's intake and output. This client is exhibiting symptoms of disseminated intravascular coagulation (DIC), and the physician should be notified. Choice **c** is incorrect. The ecchymosis was not caused by the tightness of the cuff. Rather, it is a symptom of disseminated intravascular coagulation (DIC). Choice **d** is incorrect. There is no need to retake the blood pressure at this time. The client is exhibiting symptoms of disseminated intravascular coagulation (DIC), and the physician should be notified immediately.
Category: Safe and Effective Care Environment: Management of Care
Subcategory: Maternal Infant: Maternal Complications: Postpartum

134. a. Frequent linen changes are appropriate for this client because of the diaphoresis. Diaphoresis produces general discomfort. The client should be kept dry to maintain an acceptable level of comfort. Choice **b** is incorrect. There is no indication that the client needs a bedpan. Choice **c** is incorrect. Nasotracheal suctioning is not indicated, because the client has a productive cough. Choice **d** is incorrect. The client should be repositioned every two hours.
Category: Physiological Integrity: Basic Care and Comfort
Subcategory: Adult: Respiratory Disorders

135. a. Symptoms of cocaine overdose include cardiac arrhythmias (1), increased blood pressure (2), and diarrhea (3). Choices **b**, **c**, and **d** are incorrect. Symptoms of cocaine overdose do not include pupil constriction (4).
Category: Physiological Integrity: Physiological Adaptation
Subcategory: Mental Health: Substance Abuse

136. b. The nurse is helping the client manage pain and comfort level. The nurse has completed assessment of the client and should now dim the room lights to create a quiet environment. Nonpharmacologic measures such as adjusting the lighting level in the room can facilitate pain management. Decreasing stimulation from the environment, such as brightness to the optic nerve, aids in the client's ability to relax skeletal muscles and fall asleep. Choice **a** is incorrect. There is no indication that oxygen should be administered. Choice **c** is incorrect. Checking on whether the client's family is comfortable is important, but is not higher in priority than the client's comfort. Choice **d** is incorrect. The nurse has already completed the client assessment. It is too soon to reassess the client's vital signs.
Category: Safe and Effective Care Environment: Management of Care
Subcategory: Adult: Gastrointestinal Disorders

137. c. This value is abnormal. Bleeding precautions must be initiated when the platelet count decreases. The normal platelet count is 150,000 to 450,000/mm^3. When the platelet count falls below 50,000/mm^3, any small trauma can lead to episodes of prolonged bleeding. Choice **a** is incorrect. This value is within the normal range for ammonia, which is 10 to 80 mcg/dL. Choice **b** is incorrect. This value is within the normal range for clotting time, which is 8 to 15 minutes. Choice **d** is incorrect. This value is within the normal range for white blood cell count, which is 4,500 to 11,000/mm^3.
Category: Safe and Effective Care Environment: Management of Care
Subcategory: Adult: Oncology Disorders

138. b. Each dose of sulfisoxazole should be administered with a full glass of water, and the client should maintain a high fluid intake. The medication is more soluble in alkaline urine. Choice **a** is incorrect. The client should not be instructed to taper off or discontinue the dosage of medication. Choice **c** is incorrect. Some forms of sulfisoxazole may cause urine to turn dark brown or red. This is an expected side effect and the physician does not need to be notified. Choice **d** is incorrect. The client should be instructed to maintain a high fluid intake, not to restrict fluid intake.
Category: Physiological Integrity: Pharmacological and Parenteral Therapies
Subcategory: Adult: Renal Disorders

139. c. The nurse should include the avoidance of popping an acne pimple (1), the application of topical creams (2), and the use of birth control with Accutane (4). Choices **a**, **b**, and **d** are incorrect. Sebum production (3) increases during the teen years.
Category: Health Promotion and Maintenance
Subcategory: Pediatrics: Integumentary Disorders

140. d. An injection of Tensilon makes the client in cholinergic crisis temporarily worse. Cholinergic crisis indicates an overdose of medication; thus, it is reasonable that a worsening of the condition will occur when additional medication is administered. Choice **a** is incorrect. The client experiencing cholinergic crisis would have worsening symptoms, but they would not include muscle spasms. Choice **b** is incorrect. Improvements in the client's weakness indicate myasthenic crisis. Choice **c** is incorrect. The client experiencing cholinergic crisis would have worsening of symptoms.
Category: Physiological Integrity: Pharmacological and Parenteral Therapies
Subcategory: Adult: Neurological Disorders

141. c. Increased exercise (3) and monitoring and control of the client's glucose (4) can promote increased blood flow to the brain and assist in the prevention of further cognitive changes. Choice **a** is incorrect. Aricept (1) is used to treat Alzheimer's dementia. A diet high in thiamine (2) is used to prevent Wernicke's encephalopathy in clients with alcoholism. Choice **b** is incorrect. While increased exercise (3) can increase blood flow to the brain and assist in the prevention of further cognitive changes, a diet high in thiamine (2) is used to prevent Wernicke's encephalopathy in clients with alcoholism. Choice **d** is incorrect. While monitoring and controlling the client's glucose (4) can promote increased blood flow to the brain and assist in the prevention of further cognitive changes, Aricept (1) is used to treat Alzheimer's dementia.
Category: Physiological Integrity: Reduction of Risk Potential
Subcategory: Mental Health: Cognitive Disorders

142. c. Medications 1, 2, 4, and 5 are H_2-receptor antagonists, which suppress secretions of gastric acid, alleviate symptoms of heartburn, and assist in preventing complications of peptic ulcer disease. These medications suppress gastric secretions and are prescribed for clients experiencing active ulcer disease, erosive esophagitis, and pathological hypersecretory conditions. Choice **d** is incorrect. Prevacid (3) is a protein pump inhibitor. Choices **a** and **b** are incorrect. Each does not list all the medication choices that apply.
Category: Physiological Integrity: Pharmacological and Parenteral Therapies
Subcategory: Adult: Gastrointestinal Disorders

143. c. When a client's station is +3, the fetal presenting part is 3 cm below the ischial spines. This client's fetus is furthest into the birth canal and, based only on this information, is most likely to be the first to deliver. Choice **a** is incorrect. When a client's station is 0, the fetal presenting part is at the level of the ischial spines. Choice **b** is incorrect. When a client's station is –1, the fetal presenting part is 1 cm above the ischial spines. Choice **d** is incorrect. When a client's station is –3, the fetal presenting part is 3 cm above the ischial spines.
Category: Safe and Effective Care Environment: Management of Care
Subcategory: Maternal Infant: Intrapartum

144. d. During an MRI, the client should wear no metal objects, such as jewelry, because the strong magnetic field can pull on them, causing injury to the client and, if the objects fly off, causing injury to others. Choice **a** is incorrect. The client is permitted to ask questions during the scan. The MRI scanner is equipped with a microphone. Choice **b** is incorrect. The client must lie still during the scan. Choice **c** is incorrect. The client will hear thumping sounds during the scan, which are caused by changes in the magnetic field created by the MRI machine.
Category: Safe and Effective Care Environment: Safety and Infection Control
Subcategory: Adult: Miscellaneous

145. c. The headache and irritability may be indicative of shunt malfunction, and the nurse should notify the physician of the findings. Choice **a** is incorrect. Although the nurse should document the findings, the nurse should first notify the physician, as these findings are indicative of shunt malfunction. Choice **b** is incorrect. Tylenol can be ordered for treatment of headaches. However, in this case, the headache may be indicative of shunt malfunction and therefore needs to be brought to the attention of the physician. Choice **d** is incorrect. Restraints are utilized when there is a risk of self-harm or harm to others. In this case, the irritability and combativeness and the headache may be indicative of shunt malfunction, so the physician needs to be notified.
Category: Safe and Effective Care Environment: Management of Care
Subcategory: Pediatrics: Neurological/Cognitive Disorders

146. c. The client who has a fever and is diaphoretic is the priority because this client requires comfort measures and interventions to relieve the fever. Choice **a** is incorrect. The client requiring colostomy irrigation would not take precedence over the client who has a fever and is diaphoretic. Choice **b** is incorrect. The client requiring a chest X-ray would not take precedence over the client who has a fever and is diaphoretic. Choice **d** is incorrect. The nurse should allow the pain medication to take effect before providing care for this client.
Category: Safe and Effective Care Environment: Management of Care
Subcategory: Adult: Miscellaneous

147. b. The client who is recovering from a relatively minor surgery, such as an appendectomy (2) and the client who is experiencing an exacerbation of ulcerative colitis (4) are appropriate clients to assign to an LPN, as the care they require falls within the scope of practice for an LPN. Choices **a**, **c**, and **d** are incorrect. It is not within the scope of practice for the LPN to administer TPN (1), provide client teaching related to medications (3), or insert NG tubes (5).
Category: Safe and Effective Care Environment: Management of Care
Subcategory: Adult: Miscellaneous

148. b. To help the client control episodes of hypoglycemia, the nurse should instruct the client to eat a high-protein, low-carbohydrate diet, and avoid fasting. Choice **a** is incorrect. Consuming a candy bar when feeling lightheaded will not control hypoglycemia. Choice **c** is incorrect. Increasing foods high in saturated fats and fasting in the afternoon will not control hypoglycemia. The client should also be instructed to avoid simple sugars. Choice **d** is incorrect. Taking iron and increasing foods high in vitamins B and D will not control hypoglycemia.
Category: Physiological Integrity: Basic Care and Comfort
Subcategory: Adult: Endocrine Disorders

149. a. The nurse should pull the pinna down and back. Choice **b** is incorrect. Pulling the pinna down and outward would not fully open the ear canal. Choices **c** and **d** are incorrect. Pulling the pinna up and either back or outward would obstruct entry into the ear canal.
Category: Physiological Integrity: Pharmacological and Parenteral Therapies
Subcategory: Pediatrics: Medication Administration

150. d. A surfactant is used to facilitate development of the lungs and would not be an appropriate intervention for a toddler. Choice **a** is incorrect. Antibiotics would be ordered to treat the respiratory infection. Choice **b** is incorrect. Steroids would most likely be ordered to decrease inflammation in the lungs. Choice **c** is incorrect. Bronchodilators would most likely be ordered to facilitate oxygenation.
Category: Safe and Effective Care Environment: Management of Care
Subcategory: Pediatrics: Respiratory Disorders

151. b. To convert pounds into kilograms, the nurse should divide the weight in pounds by 2.2; 62 divided by 2.2 is 28.18. The nurse should document the child's weight as 28.18 kg. Choice **a** is incorrect. To convert pounds into kilograms, the nurse should divide the weight in pounds by 2.2, not 2.3. Choice **c** is incorrect. To convert pounds into kilograms, the nurse should divide, not multiply, the child's weight by 2.2; 62 divided by 2.2 is 28.18. Choice **d** is incorrect. To convert pounds into kilograms, the nurse should divide the child's weight by 2.2, not multiply by 2.22. The nurse should not round.
Category: Health Promotion and Maintenance
Subcategory: Pediatrics: Assessment

152. b. The nurse should always respect the client's cultural beliefs (4) and ask if the client has cultural or religious requirements (1); this may include food choices or restrictions, body coverings, or time for prayer. Nonverbal cues may have different meanings in different cultures (5). In one culture, eye contact is a sign of disrespect; in another, eye contact shows respect and attentiveness. Choices **a**, **c**, and **d** are incorrect. The nurse should attempt to understand the client's culture; the client does not need to understand the nurse's culture (2), and nurses should never impose their own beliefs on clients. Culture influences a client's experience with pain (3); not all cultures experience or describe pain in the same way.
Category: Psychosocial Integrity
Subcategory: Adult: Miscellaneous

153. b. Clients with depersonalization disorder may experience feeling detached from the body. Choice **a** is incorrect. Hallucinations occur with dissociative identity disorder. Choice **c** is incorrect. Memory loss is associated with dissociative amnesia. Choice **d** is incorrect. While anxiety can be a symptom of many types of mental illness, it is not a symptom of depersonalization disorder.
Category: Physiological Integrity: Physiological Adaptation
Subcategory: Mental Health: Personality Disorders

154. b. It is important for the nurse to assess this client for dysphasia. Radiation-induced esophagitis with dysphasia is rather common in clients who received radiation to the chest. The anatomic location of the esophagus is posterior to the mediastinum and is within the field of primary treatment. Choice **a** is incorrect. Diarrhea is uncommon in the treatment of lung cancer. Choice **c** is incorrect. Decreased energy level is a potential complication of radiation therapy. Choice **d** is incorrect. Decreased white blood cell count is a potential complication of radiation therapy.
Category: Physiological Integrity: Reduction of Risk Potential
Subcategory: Adult: Oncology Disorders

155. c. Clients with Addison's disease will experience decreased hepatic gluconeogenesis and increased tissue glucose uptake, which causes hypoglycemia. Choice **a** is incorrect. Clients with Addison's disease will experience an elevated BUN level. There is a decrease in excretion of waste products. Choice **b** is incorrect. Clients with Addison's disease will experience hyponatremia, not hypernatremia. Choice **d** is incorrect. Clients with Addison's disease will experience hyperkalemia, not hypocalcemia.
Category: Physiological Integrity: Reduction of Risk Potential
Subcategory: Adult: Endocrine Disorders

156. a. Mongolian spots appear as blue to slate gray marks on an infant's buttocks, back, and legs. While they may resemble bruising, they are a benign color variation that will usually disappear by two years of age. Mongolian spots are common among darker-skinned persons, such as those who are of Asian, East Indian, and African descent. Choice **b** is incorrect. Montgomery spots appear as white spots on the areola of a pregnant/nursing woman. Choice **c** is incorrect. The nurse is observing Mongolian spots, which are a benign color variation; therefore, notifying the physician is inappropriate at this time. Choice **d** is incorrect. The nurse is observing Mongolian spots, which appear as blue to slate-grey marks on an infant's buttocks, back, and legs. While they may resemble bruising, they are a benign color variation that will usually disappear by two years of age.
Category: Health Promotion and Maintenance
Subcategory: Maternal Infant: Neonate Assessment

157. a. Sudden, severe abdominal pain can be indicative of placental abruption, which is the premature separation of the placenta from the uterus. Choice **b** is incorrect. A client with eclampsia would experience elevated blood pressure, protein in the urine, and seizures, but not abdominal pain and dark red vaginal bleeding. Choice **c** is incorrect. A client with HELLP syndrome would experience upper abdominal pain, changes in vision, and nausea and vomiting, but not dark red vaginal bleeding. Choice **d** is incorrect. The client with placenta previa would experience painless vaginal bleeding, usually bright red in color.
Category: Safe and Effective Care Environment: Management of Care
Subcategory: Maternal Infant: Maternal Complications: Intrapartum

158. d. The nurse should assess the client's cognition (2) and utilize relaxation techniques (4). Choice **a** is incorrect. The use of chemical restraints (1) is not appropriate at this time, as there is no indication that the client is at risk for harming self or others. Choices **b** and **c** are incorrect. The nurse should ensure a nonstimulating environment for the client, rather than one that provides stimulation (3).
Category: Psychosocial Integrity
Subcategory: Mental Health: Cognitive Disorders

159. b. Diplegia is the term used when the dysfunction is greater in the lower extremities. Choice **a** is incorrect. Quadriplegia is the term utilized when the dysfunction is equal in all four extremities. Choice **c** is incorrect. In diplegic cerebral palsy, the dysfunction is greater in the lower extremities. Choice **d** is incorrect. Hemiplegia is the term utilized when the dysfunction involves only one side of the body.
Category: Physiological Integrity: Basic Care and Comfort
Subcategory: Pediatrics: Neurological/ Cognitive Disorders

160. d. During the taking-hold phase, the mother feels more in control and is ready to focus on learning how to care for her infant. Choice **a** is incorrect. Symptoms of depression usually surface during Rubin's letting-go phase. Choice **b** is incorrect. The taking-hold phase is an appropriate time to conduct client education. Contacting the physician to perform a circumcision on the infant is inappropriate at this time. Choice **c** is incorrect. The client should be encouraged to verbalize her birthing experience during the taking-in phase, not the taking-hold phase.
Category: Psychosocial Integrity
Subcategory: Maternal Infant: Postpartum

161. d. Clients with acute pancreatitis are at risk for developing complications associated with the respiratory system. Atelectasis, pneumonia, and pleural effusions are some examples of complications that can develop as a result of pancreatic enzyme exudate. Choices **a**, **b**, and **c** are incorrect. Acute pancreatitis does not cause any of these conditions.
Category: Physiological Integrity: Reduction of Risk Potential
Subcategory: Adult: Gastrointestinal Disorders

162. d. The client should be instructed to wear loose clothing to protect extremities from the cold. Wearing gloves when handling cold objects will help prevent vasospasms. Choice **a** is incorrect. Elevating the hands and feet as much as possible is contraindicated, as this will decrease arterial perfusion during periods of vasospasms. Choice **b** is incorrect. The client should be taught to avoid caffeine as well as tobacco. Choice **c** is incorrect. The client should be instructed not to use vibrating equipment, as this contributes to the production of vasospasms.
Category: Safe and Effective Care Environment: Management of Care
Subcategory: Adult: Cardiovascular Disorders

163. c. When dehiscence occurs, the nurse should immediately cover the wound with a sterile dressing moistened with normal saline. If the dehiscence is extensive, the client may be returned to surgery to be resutured. Choice **a** is incorrect. Applying an abdominal binder may be appropriate, but it is not what the nurse should do immediately. Choice **b** is incorrect. After the sutures are removed, not before, additional support may be provided to the incision by applying strips of tape as ordered by the surgeon. Choice **d** is incorrect. Irrigating the wound with sterile water is not an appropriate nursing intervention.
Category: Physiological Integrity: Reduction of Risk Potential
Subcategory: Adult: Gastrointestinal Disorders

164. a. Proximodistal refers to growth from the center of the body outward. The arms are located closer to the center of the body than the fingers, so the child will gain control of arm movement before finger movement. Choice **b** is incorrect. Control of arm then leg movement is an example of cephalocaudal, or head-to-feet, growth. Choice **c** is incorrect. Proximodistal refers to growth from the center of the body outward. The arms are located closer to the center of the body than the fingers, so the child will gain control of arm movement before finger movement. Choice **d** is incorrect. According to the growth and development principle of cephalocaudal growth (head to-feet growth) the child will gain control of arm then leg movement.

Category: Physiological Integrity: Basic Care and Comfort

Subcategory: Pediatrics: Growth and Development Theories

165. c. The period of preoperational thought occurs in children two to seven years old and is characterized by attributing life to inanimate objects, use of pretend play, and seeing the self as the center of the world. Choice **a** is incorrect. The period of concrete operational thought occurs in children ages seven to 12 years old and is characterized by focusing on the present and a realistic understanding of the world. Choice **b** is incorrect. The period of formal operational thought occurs in children over the age of 12 and is characterized by the ability to think abstractly. Choice **d** is incorrect. The sensorimotor period occurs in children zero to two years old and is characterized by an understanding of night and day, object permanence, and cause and effect.

Category: Physiological Integrity: Basic Care and Comfort

Subcategory: Pediatrics: Growth and Development Theories

ADDITIONAL ONLINE PRACTICE

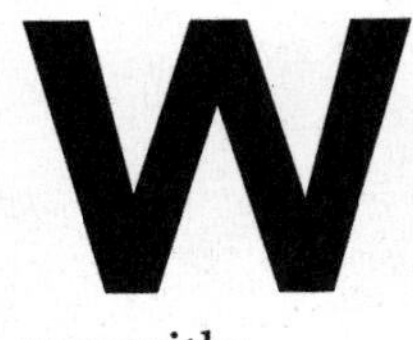

hether you need help building basic skills or preparing for an exam, visit the LearningExpress Practice Center! On this site, you can access additional practice materials. Using the code below, you'll be able to log in and take an additional practice test. This online practice will also provide you with:

- **Immediate scoring**
- **Detailed answer explanations**
- **Personalized recommendations for further practice and study**

Log in to the LearningExpress Practice Center by using this URL: **www.learnatest.com/practice**

This is your Access Code: **9087**

Follow the steps online to redeem your access code. After you've used your access code to register with the site, you will be prompted to create a username and password. For easy reference, record them here:

Username: ____________________ **Password:** ____________________

With your username and password, you can log in and access your additional practice materials. If you have any questions or problems, please contact LearningExpress customer service at 1-800-295-9556 ext. 2, or e-mail us at **customerservice@learningexpressllc.com.**